Superior Health

The Secrets Of The Chinese And Eastern Way

Superior Health

The Secrets Of The Chinese And Eastern Way

By

Myles Wray

To Lisa,

Wishing you Health And Happiness,

Myles Wray

The information contained in this book has been gathered from reliable sources. However it is intended as a guide only and should not be used as a replacement for consultation with your Western or Chinese medical doctor. The reader should consult his or her medical professional before attempting any of the suggestions in this book or drawing inferences from it. All matters regarding your health require medical supervision. If you know or suspect that you have a health problem, then seek the advice of a trained health professional.

No responsibility for loss, damage or injury acting on or refraining from action as a result of the use and application of the information contained within, can be accepted by the author or publisher. The author and publisher disclaim any and all liability arising directly and indirectly from the use of any information contained within this book.

By reading this publication, the reader agrees to the terms of this disclaimer and further waives any rights or claims he or she may have against the publisher or author.

Contents

Section - 3 - Food And Diet

Section - 4 - Breathing

Section - 5 - Cancer

Section - 10 - Modern Problems

Section - 11 - Emotions And The Mind

Section - 12 - Recap And Summary

Foreword.

This book is essentially about creating a better, healthier, happier life and future for yourself through Eastern health methods and philosophies. In particular we will discuss in detail Chinese Medicine, which is the biggest, most structured Eastern system.

In the East they have many different and unique ways to cultivate health. Even their idea of what constitutes good health is quite different to our Western viewpoint. To those in the East, to be seen as healthy, you must be so on every level. The body, the mind and the spirit must all be strong and in harmony.

One of the greatest strengths of Chinese Medicine is its methods to deal with the prevention of illness. Its aim is to empower the body with such energy and vitality that no internal weakness can create an illness, nor any external disease penetrate it.

This book has been written for everyday people to give them all the information they need to understand the essential ideas and basics of this wonderful form of medicine. It is filled with practical ways that people can easily adopt and immediately start to bring into their lives.

I have tried to make this book as simple, straight forward and easy to understand as possible. When I started practicing Chinese medicine in Ireland, I often found that people in our Western society, due to our upbringing, education and culture, would sometimes find it difficult to grasp these foreign concepts. So over many years I developed a more Westernised style of explaining the structures of Chinese Medicine. I would often use Western science and its ideas to back up the theories the Chinese had formulated over the last several thousand years. In this book you will find a slightly different version to the more traditional one used in China. However it does still relate faithfully to classical formulas and principles designed by ancient and modern masters. I feel the most important thing is to get these really valuable Eastern ideas across in a way that Western minds can accept and understand. To further back up the theories of Chinese Medicine, I have included a large quantity of Western scientific trials and studies within many of the chapters. These studies reflect similar views to the Eastern visions of life and health.

We are about to begin a very rewarding journey that Western minds have never made before. As we travel down this road we will encounter many new thoughts and ideas. One thing you will need for this, is an open mind. In the West we can often be very stubborn and close minded with our beliefs. As we grow up we are surrounded by computers, space rockets, satellites and many other scientific marvels. As we are immersed in this we tend to become a little dazzled by it and assume that Western science knows it all. That it could not possibly be missing anything. And if it was, it would be the only one capable of discovering how to resolve things. When I began learning Chinese Medicine my mind was exactly like that. But after dwelling on the indisputable logic of Eastern ideas and after witnessing some astonishing changes in myself and others I have treated, my mind now fully embraces these ways. I hope that by the time you get to the end of this book you will feel the same way too.

The last big influence from the East was martial arts. Before the great martial artist Bruce Lee arrived in America in the 1970's, everyone in the West taught the ultimate ways of combat were boxing and wrestling. Eastern art forms like Kung Fu and Karate radically changed all that. Now it's hard to find an American or European action movie or television show that does not incorporate them. Boxing and wrestling have been somewhat left behind. Having mostly been replaced by the Eastern ways which have now become the main styles of combat.

There is still so much more to be learnt from China, India and the East. Particularly in the areas of physical, mental and spiritual health. If we can keep our minds open and don't dismiss things off hand before we have had a real chance to think about them, then we can often make great leaps forward in our ways of understanding life. Hopefully in the future, the brilliant and profound wisdom and insights in Chinese medicine will have an even bigger impact in the West than martial arts did. And perhaps we may see at some stage a blending of both Eastern and Western medicines, to form one great world medicine.

Introduction.

The Modern World - Something's Gone Wrong.

Over the last seventy years, the face of disease has significantly changed. People used to suffer from diseases of poverty, of not having enough of the essentials. From lack of food and nutrients, and other basics like heat and shelter in cold winters, to lack of clean water and poor or no sanitation to prevent the spread of germs. This led to illnesses like pneumonia, lung problems, rheumatic heart disease, infections, tuberculosis, measles and problems relating to pregnancy and childbirth. People simply had too little to keep their bodies strong and healthy.

Nowadays the pendulum has swung to the other side. People are suffering from diseases of affluence. Of having too much food, indulgences and even desires. In particular the last thirty years has seen major escalations in degenerative diseases such as obesity, type 2 diabetes, heart disease, cancer, strokes, high cholesterol, depression, high blood pressure, dementia, Alzheimer's, and allergies. The list goes on and on, with new diseases often being added. Our modern world seems to be weakening us, to be making us sick, to be diminishing our standard of living and our ability for real joy and happiness. It even seems to be killing off many of us prematurely.

Our economies and healthcare systems are coming under increasing threat. Facing an escalating burden from the rising costs of treatments from the ever growing numbers of ill people. Some governments are even discussing the possibility of their healthcare systems going bankrupt if something is not done to reign in these enlarging numbers. Our Western medical system after promising so much seems to be lost and struggling to keep up with modern problems. It does not appear to be effective in producing a decline in health issues. And what it does give seems to come at both a high financial cost and often in regard to side effects, an even higher price to many of us in terms of the rest of our health and quality of life. The average age of the chronically ill and people who have become dependant on Western drugs is becoming younger and younger with each passing decade. Even many of our children are already lined up for lives of pill popping. Large numbers of them are now hooked on behavioural medicines such as anti-depressants and drugs for attention deficit hyperactivity disorder. The latest statistics show that nearly one in five young American adults has some form of personality disorder.

Indeed, there seems to be ever increasing ways in which modern living can harm us. Between pollutants and chemicals in our food and environment, to the constant barrage of negativity from the news and media, to the breakdown of our communities and families and the isolation of our hearts and souls. Our society is clearly heading in the wrong direction.

The deep human connections we need to keep our souls strong seem to be fading away. More than fifty percent of all US marriages now end in divorce, damaging not just millions of adults but their children as well. A third of all US births are to single mothers. Families are truly in the decline.

Real friendships people used to have are now being replaced by undependable distant acquaintances on the internet. Our elderly too are becoming more isolated within society. They are suffering from more physical and mental disabilities at earlier and earlier ages. The levels of dementia and Alzheimer's are increasing at what can only be described as astounding rates. Many of the elderly now live their remaining years alone and suffering mental and emotional neglect in care institutions and hospitals.

Our lives too have become so rushed and stressed that we no longer have any time for meaningful connections. Our culture and media bombard us daily with unobtainable dreams, we must have this, we must have that, or according to them we will suffer and lead empty and worthless lives. We seem now to be just trying to live an 'image' rather than a happy, contented, joyful, loving life. The amount of strain and pressure on the human mind has caused frightening increases in the levels of depression and mental illness. One of the main factors leading to this is the loneliness and sense of disconnection many of us now feel in the modern world. We can clearly see that the relationship between health and modern living is very closely tied from what has happened in India, China and other developing nations. As they have become more Westernised, adopting Western processed foods and styles of living, their levels of killer and debilitating diseases have also skyrocketed at alarming rates.

So it is time for a change. Now we can wait for Western Medicine and mainstream society to change (which might be an awfully long wait). Or we can take matters into our own hands and begin to change ourselves. We don't need to do anything too radical, we don't need to abandon science and technology and go back to living in caves and forests. We just need to start thinking a little bit more deeply and become aware of what's really important to us. We need to become wiser and more selective about what is useful and what is not in all areas of our lives. From our personal lives to what we take on board from our science, culture and media.

Some parts of technology have been great for the world. Many advancements have clearly raised standards of living and have made things easier for us in lots of ways. Many improvements have saved lives, increased communications and knowledge. It is indeed thanks to the internet and our modern communication methods that I have been able to research and learn so much in order to write this book. However the same technology that has given us so much, has also caused destruction and pollution on a massive scale. Everything from Global Warming to the creation of numerous new illnesses. Many would also say that as it has grown, it has weakened the value of life and diminished the place for our souls in this world. We need to refocus our technology to work with nature and indeed with ourselves.

In this book we will learn techniques which can help us to change for the better. And hopefully as we change, we may influence society to come along with us. These methods are not difficult to learn but initially they do require a little bit of effort and persistence. If you follow them patiently you will see not just your physical health improve, but your emotions and entire life will too.

When all is said and done, life is about happiness and nothing else. Power, wealth and fame, although they seem very desirable have proven themselves time and time again not to lead to fulfilment and lasting happiness. There are endless examples of Hollywood stars, singers, celebrities and wealthy business tycoons who seem to have it all, to be living the dream. And yet daily we hear and read about the many problems and illnesses they suffer from. Depression, anxiety, cancers and heart attacks seem to be as common in their worlds as ours.

You will find that when you become healthy in the right way through Eastern Medicine, that this real health will significantly increase your levels of happiness, regardless of most circumstances in your personal life. You will find also as your mind clears, that many of the problems you face on a daily basis don't seem to be so troubling anymore and with this new clarity you can quickly and easily deal with such issues. There are so many simple and easy practices we can include in our daily lives which will bring us closer to our goal of happiness. A healthy body and a healthy mental perspective will also nourish our deepest essence, our souls. Our health and happiness is truly in our hands.

Some alarming statistics relating to health in our modern world are given below. When you read them do bear in mind how quickly the diseases are escalating over such short periods of time …

The 2009 World Alzheimer's Report estimates 35 million people are now living with Alzheimer's and dementia, an increase of 10 percent since 2005.

A report from the London School Of Economics and the Institute Of Psychiatry projects current figures of 700,000 people with dementia in the UK will jump to over 1.7 million by 2051. While Alzheimer's Australia estimates figures will leap from 245,000 dementia sufferers currently to 1.3 million by 2051. And The Alzheimer's Society of Scotland predicts cases of dementia will rise from 58,000 to 102,000 by 2031.

The Lancet Medical Journal issued a report predicting an alarming increase of blood pressure cases to rise from 972 million in 2000 to an estimate of 1.56 billion by 2025.

The National Academy of Sciences Institute Of Medicine issued a report claiming a 30 percent increase in premature births in the US since 1981. Premature babies are at a much greater risk for many illnesses throughout their lives.

According to UK government statistics oral cancer has increased by 53 percent between 1997 and 2007. Liver cancer by 43 percent over the same period. Breast cancer by 33 percent and colorectal cancer by 14 percent. Between 1997 and 2006 the UK government has also reported an increase of 120 percent in cases of bowel cancer among the under thirties.

The world Health Organization expects global cancer cases to reach 27 million by 2030. It states that cancer rates jumped from 5.9 million in 1975 to 12 million in 2007.

A report from Teresa Seeman and others in UCLA found that various disabilities in 60 to 69 year olds had risen by up to 70 percent between 1988 and 2004. Difficulties in such everyday routines like walking, eating, dressing, house work and cooking.

The Archives of General Psychiatry released a study stating that 1 in 5 young people between 19 and 25 in the US now has a personality disorder.

According to the Centres for Disease Control in the US, 10 percent of children between 12 and 17 are now medicated for attention deficit hyperactivity disorder.

The Australian Bureau of Statistics reported a 9 percent increase in mental ill health between 2005 and 2008. It also reported a staggering 26 percent of young people aged between 16 and 24 had some form of mental illness in 2007.

The UK government estimates 10 percent of UK children now have a clinically recognisable mental disorder.

The Journal of Child Psychology and Psychiatry reports that almost 15 percent of preschoolers now have abnormally high levels of anxiety and depression.

From 1997 to 2003 the UK government reported an increase of 74 percent of new cases of type 2 diabetes.

The Australian Institute of Health and Welfare reported an increase of 26 percent in Kidney diseases between 2000 and 2007.

Skin Cancer rates rose by 50 percent in men over a period of ten years from 1996 to 2006 in Scotland according to government figures.

The UK Government body Foresight predicts that 60 percent of UK men and 50 percent of women will be obese by 2050. While a study in the Journal Obesity predicts that 86 percent of Americans will be obese by 2030. The figure currently stands at 66 percent.

A paper in the Journal of the Royal Society of Medicine reports an increase of 42 percent in cases of eczema in the UK between 2001 and 2005.

Section One - The Background And Theories Of Eastern Medicine.

Chapter One - What Is Real Health ?

In the West, health is usually defined as the absence of illness. That is to say, the absence of any diseased or mutating cells or the presence of any unfriendly bacteria or viruses. Good health is often portrayed as being physically fit. Your ability to run quickly or over long distances or to do press ups and so forth is seen as a primary indicator of your good health. In regard to the mind, as long as you are not clinically depressed, the absence of joy and good spirits is not deemed necessary for health. And as for our souls, they don't even get a passing nod to their existence and needs.

These days many people can no longer even recognize what good health should be. Even when they exercise daily and have apparently fit and disease free bodies, they accept tiredness, anxiety, frustration, poor sleep, mood swings and feeling low as normal ways of livings. I was one of these people until I found Chinese Medicine.

The description in Asia for health is very different. Someone is not considered healthy if they just have a fit body, but instead they need to be mentally, emotionally, physically and spiritually well to have the claim of real full health. The spirit cannot be excluded and alienated from the body. The spirit is the fundamental core of our body and existence. If our spirit has become weak and starved of meaning then this will eventually lead to a poor state of mind which weakens the body and will inevitably lead to illness. A healthy person should feel fresh, full of endless energy and happy to be alive. Their minds should be bright and clear. They should easily be able to cope with and bounce back from any knocks and troubles life throws at them. They should have vibrant radiant health allowing them to make the most productive outcomes of their time here on earth.

Chinese Medicine is also concerned not just with avoiding ills and feeling good now, but ensuring that the body has strong reserves built up for it to continue to have strength and joy in old age. A healthy person should not suffer from arthritis, frailty, diminished mobility, loss of cognitive and mental functioning, heart disease and other Western geriatric ills. We should instead have a sharp mind and memory, a limber body and strength and health which allows us to continue a fulfilling life right through our elderly years. In China and Asia there are many who continue working into their eighties and even nineties, who have rewarding lives being able to help their families and communities. And in return receiving love and respect back from them.

You will find many great tools in this book to give you real health. Obviously the more of them that you do and bring into your life on a daily basis, the more you will get back.

As there is quite a lot to learn and change from current Western ways of living, you can start with just a few basics. And over time you will be able to add more and more of them without any difficulty, until you have incorporated most of these methods into your life. Every time you do add one of these ways, you will be rewarded by seeing and feeling the good changes and benefits they create.

Because there is such a substantial amount of information in this book, it is a wise idea to keep a pen beside it as you are reading. Then you can mark any areas of interest, so you can easily be able to reread and reference them as you start to apply these new techniques and ways to your life.

Chapter Two - What Is So Special About Eastern Ways ?

Chinese Medicine is filled with abundant free and low cost, easy and proven methods of not just restoring but with a little time and effort giving you peak radiant health. Health that you and every other human being deserve to have. It is logical and full of common sense and practical helpful ways to immediately help you start improving your life. It is also very easy to follow and utilize.

As I was growing up I was led to believe that most illnesses were solely down to pure bad luck, you caught this or that. Nowadays, your genes which are seen like a lottery, will supposedly give you this or that, taking all responsibility for your future out of your hands. But when I studied Chinese Medicine those ideas quickly fell apart, not only could I see how health and illness were very clearly the product of how you lived your life, but I could also see exactly the things I had done to cause the problems I had. And fortunately for me, it had now taught me all I needed to resolve every last one of them.

Chinese Medicine gives you the knowledge and with that comes freedom and independence. It teaches us how to utilize the incredible power we have inside our own bodies to bring about health and happiness. All it takes is to follow the steps and in time we can become masters of our own health, harmony and destiny.

Chapter Three - The Miracle Of The Human Body.

The human body is quite simply incredible. Its ability to regenerate and its potential to heal when given the right conditions is simply outstanding. It is by all accounts, a living breathing marvel.

So what makes it so special ?

For starters the body grows from a few cells into a baby, then a child, then a teenager and finally into an adult all by itself with very little help or interference. There is nothing even close in science that can perform such a miracle.

An adult body is composed of about five billion billion billion atoms. Which make one hundred trillion cells. All of which know exactly what to do and are working away right now keeping your body and mind in shape. There are about fifty thousand miles of blood vessels in a body. That's about twice the circumference of the world. Your brain has about one hundred billion nerve cells which form our thoughts and memories. Inside it, there is a maze of electrical signals just like in a computer. However, your brain can and does rewire its circuits when it needs to. Even after a stroke, your brain given the right circumstances can move functions from damaged parts and restart them in healthier ones. The rest of our nerve cells make up a complete system. A kind of wire circuitry around the body. These allow electrical signals to race around the body at around four hundred kilometres an hour. As for our hearts, they beat on average one hundred thousand times a day. Leading to a whopping three billion times over an average life span.

Some of its greatest feats are to do with regeneration. The body is constantly replacing its cells, tissues and organs. Our livers will replace every cell, giving you a brand new one over a period of about three to five months. Some of the cells in your lungs replace themselves every two to three weeks. Your entire lungs will be replaced over the space of about a year. Your skin sheds itself and is replaced every two to four weeks. Some cells in the intestine regenerate and help to build new linings every two to five days. Even your bones will be fully replaced with a new set every ten years.

Our bodies are truly a masterpiece. They are composed of energy, matter, mind and soul. And although science is great at many things, as it can break down, observe and isolate our bodies into smaller and smaller fragments, there is however a lot it still cannot achieve. It can interfere with existing life but essentially cannot create life itself. And as for the soul, it simply has no real understanding of it at all. It has never been able to expand on the issue of the soul. So it simply chooses to ignore it and yet we all know without doubt that we have one.

When it comes to health, many of us are living our lives in the dark. Unaware of our massive capabilities and potential to heal. The body often gives hints of these powers in the way it can heal itself from coughs, colds, flu, cuts, bruises and broken bones with little or no intervention at all. When we stop polluting our bodies with cigarettes and too much alcohol, with toxic food and stress, we begin to see remarkable changes in them. And in organs such as our lungs and livers. If we haven't scarred them up too badly, then much of the damage starts to reverse over six months to a year. This can produce healthy functioning organs again. Unfortunately Western education and culture has led us to believe that medical experts are the only ones who can save us. And even with their help, we are still destined to grow sickly in old age. Later in this book you will see how wrong that philosophy is.

Our bodies are designed to heal themselves, to constantly renew cells and to rebuild tissue and organs. Unless we keep causing harm to them by inappropriate behaviour, our bodies will mostly heal themselves up. And if we actually create environments that feed and nourish them, we will be amazed by how healthy we can become.

Chapter Four - The History And Evolution Of Chinese Medicine.

The reason behind including a chapter on history in this book is not to bore you but to help you understand just how big, well thought out, elaborate and scientific Chinese Medicine is.

A look at its history starts to show us why we should have great faith in it and take it so seriously. Why it stands head and shoulders above many other forms of medicine.

For starters, it has been around for thousands and thousands of years and has constantly grown and developed. It has been tested and retested over and over again throughout all this time, making it incredibly safe. It has delivered a very productive and effective method not just of curing illness, but a complete system to prevent it and also to enhance health and well being.

Chinese Medicine which is used in China and many other Eastern nations around it, is the oldest and longest continuous medical system that the world has ever known. It has successfully served generation after generation of Asian peoples for literally thousands of years. Considering that today, there are 1,300 million people in China, if you multiply this by all their ancestors for at least the last five thousand years, then you start to come up with staggering figures of the amount of people treated by Chinese Medicine. Add into that all the other countries who have used it in the past. And also include the estimated forty percent of the worlds' population who are currently using it now and you will come up with colossal figures. Even Western Medicine compares quite poorly to this. Many of its modern procedures and drugs quite often simply do not have any historical back up of proven efficacy behind them. In fact, they are sometimes using today's population as guinea pigs, completely unaware of possible long term future side effects and repercussions. This is commonly and repeatedly seen by the large number of modern drugs constantly being taken off the market, year after year, on the discovery of potentially damaging and even lethal side effects.

Why is it so important that all these people have been and are still using Chinese medicine. Well, because quite simply, anything dangerous such as toxic herbs, improper techniques or invalid theories, have all been taken out of it. Making it, when proper practices are followed, the safest established medical system in use in the world today. Not alone is it safe, but the experience gained over thousands of years on exercise, breathing, meditation, diet and other health methods is quite simply invaluable in its insights, accuracy and correct theoretical foundations.

So how did it all begin ? Well, excavations have discovered needles made from shards of stone and bones dating as far back to about seven or eight thousand years ago. The earliest recovered medical text, still in existence is the Shen Nong Ben Cao Jing from before 300 B.C. This book described in detail the use of a remarkable 365 medicinal herbal drugs and prescribed over 170 types of remedies for different illnesses. The Yellow Emperors Inner Classic, The Huang Di Nei Jing, from around 200 B.C., gave the basics of Chinese Medicine. This book is considered by modern historians to be a collection of all available knowledge relating to Chinese Medicine that had been gathered at that time and also many centuries before. By the seventh century, Chao Yuan Feng, edited the classic Pathology Of Diseases, which referred to the causes, symptoms and treatments of over 1,700 different illnesses. In 1578, the famous Chinese physician, Li Shizhen, after a near lifetime whopping 27 years of hard work and dedication, finished compiling The Compendium Of Materia Medica. It listed the uses of 1,892 medicinal substances and covered over an amazing 10,000 medical prescriptions for different ailments. All in all, before the 1900's, there have been more than 6,000 medical text books written during the great history of Chinese Medicine.

Without modern scientific methods, microscopes, computers, gadgets and technology, how did they manage to discover so much about life and disease ? Well they were not so much interested in the physiology of the human body, they were more interested in how everything reacted with everything else. And they spent thousands of years, observing and cataloguing exactly how it all fits together. You will see in the following chapters, that once you have observed and broken down the basic foundations of life and nature, it is not that difficult to come to many important conclusions on our health. And from there to keep advancing the system to higher and higher levels of wisdom and understanding. Of course it definitely helps when you throw the thoughts of geniuses like Li Shizhen and Shen Nong into the mix. And not forgetting the many physicians who by experimenting on themselves by eating herbs and minerals were able to have first hand experience of what these natural elements did. There was such dedication by these men and women, that many of them in early times, lost their own lives through poisoning from experimenting with dangerous herbs and minerals.

These masters of ancient times studied everything. From human beings to every part of nature, from life in good health to life in illness. From tasting and experimenting with herbs and foods, to studying how certain emotions tended to cause certain illnesses. To the effects of the weather on people and animals. And even to animal themselves. How they moved, reacted, their strengths, abilities and weaknesses. How some of them like cats, turtles and monkeys even stood in meditative like poses, bathing in the sun and taking advantage of its warm energies. And after observing all that, they would gather, collect, share and log all these facts, developing their own scientific theories along the way. When they treated patients, they noted not just the illnesses but also any other characteristics the person displayed as well. Such as the way they looked, talked, behaved and even noting if there were any body odours from them.

Over time by correlating all these details they were able to build up patterns that diseases fitted into. For example, an angry, agitated, red faced, hot individual might often suffer from thumping headaches, or be prone to high pitched ringing in his ears or have an unusually high chance of suffering a stroke. The underlying pattern here causing all these problems is stemming from too much heat, internal pressure and stress. The solution in this case is to simply give the patient acupuncture or herbs and lifestyle advice to help cool and relax them, bringing their body back into balance. This sounds very simple, but as you will learn, the Chinese have more than proven that simplicity works and works really well. Quite often life and good health are really not that complicated at all. The only ones who want to make it so are those who want to deceive you of your hard earned money. They are very clever and good at keeping you ignorant and in the dark, so you can't see the truth and help fix yourself without them.

The emperors and rulers of China also had a pivotal role to play in the formation of Chinese Medicine. They had incredible power and wealth. They had lives of luxury and splendour, filled with fine foods, art, music, entertainment, riches and leisure. In order to maximise their enjoyment of all this, many searched for longevity and even immortality. They constantly sent their physicians to all corners of China to gather information and knowledge to help them in this quest. This helped to build up an incredibly vast library and well maintained network of knowledge, which was shared right across China in the treatment and prevention of illness and of course the many methods to enhance life and to live strong and healthy into and throughout old age.

However emperors and physicians of China were not alone. Along with them, religious and spiritual orders and philosophies had a great input into the development of Chinese Medicine.

Confucius (551 - 479 B.C.), was a moral teacher who formed and developed an ethical and philosophical system based on the ethics and politics of good behaviour. The basic principle was to develop the people morally so that society could be governed not by coercive laws but by moral virtues. He taught many things, including that the young needed to be nurtured by society and that the elderly needed to be respected and have a fulfilling existence until they departed from this world. Everything was done to promote a meaningful and harmonious society. The legacy of this system existed in China until the early 1900's. This obviously had profound effects on the values of physicians in the treatment of patients and in their own desires to help make a better society. Such was the moral responsibilities which went with being a doctor that many were only paid when they kept their clients well. This ensured they were doing their best and gave them great incentive to get anyone who became ill better again as quickly as possible. I wonder how much Western Medicine would quickly change and improve if such a system was introduced in our present times.

Buddhism was said to be brought to China from India. From it many methods of meditation were developed to lead its practitioners towards a state of Nirvana - a state of pure bliss, joy, peace and happiness. One of the principles of Buddhism is compassion to fellow human beings. And many Buddhists who devised ways of keeping themselves fit and healthy for their spiritual practices, willingly shared these methods with the communities they were a part of.

The last major religious philosophy in China is Daoism. It is based on the Dao, translated as The Way. The Way was to try and live a balanced and harmonious life with nature, existence and fellow humans, rather than to constantly try to manipulate things and struggle against them. The Daoists were particularly interested in achieving longevity and even immortality. They meditated, exercised and studied nature, experimenting with herbs, potions, and elixirs in their efforts to achieve this. Many Daoists shared their discoveries with fellow practitioners and those interested in Daoism.

The result of the influence of Confucianism, Buddhism and Daoism on Chinese Medicine was to create a medical system that was devised on genuine spiritual and philosophical beliefs. On truly doing what was in the best and most compassionate interests of the patient and the general well being and improvement of all of society. Hippocrates, credited as the original founding father of Western Medicine, had similar values and ideals way back in ancient Greece. However, today, it is often very clear that for many involved in modern Western Medicine, money and not compassion nor quality care for patients has become the main motivational factor. This unfortunately has not just hurt the patient but also all the good doctors out there, who strive to improve the Western Medical system.

In more modern history of China, since the Chinese Revolution of 1949, the Communist government has repeatedly tested all aspects of Chinese Medicine. They concluded, after performing thousands of tests, trials and clinical studies, that it is a very valid and productive form of medicine. And without any doubt whatsoever, it works very effectively. In China, they have given it an equal place with Western Medicine. There are many hospitals which specialize in

Chinese Medicine alone. And in most other modern hospitals, you will find a mix of Chinese and Western Medicines. You may typically find someone who receives Western surgery will then recuperate with Chinese herbs and Medical Qi Gong exercises.

As you can see through its magnificent history, Chinese Medicine clearly stands alone in the vast and impressive quantity of empirical evidence and refined theories created and collected on billions and billions of people over thousands and thousands of years. Its moral ethics and desire to genuinely improve life is unquestionable. It is not by just luck and chance that there are more Chinese than any other race on the earth but a true measure of the incredible techniques and life enhancing methods of Chinese Medicine and its philosophies.

Chapter Five - The Big Picture.

In the following chapters we will start to see what practical Chinese Medicine is all about. But before that we need to understand some of its basic principles and theories before we can make use of them to strengthen our everyday lives.

This part of the book may not be overly interesting to some readers. But it is necessary to give the background and basics needed to enable you to make good use of Chinese Medicine. If you are patient and read through the more difficult parts, you will be rewarded by all the more interesting and clever stuff in the later parts of the book.

Let's begin with the big picture. Asians take a very different view of the world than we do in the West. If we were both asked to look at the same picture of a man in front of a building, the Western mind set is usually to focus in on the man in explicit detail. However, the Eastern mind would instead focus on the background and entire picture including the man. Our Western minds and upbringing have geared us towards concentrating in on small details and fine points. But sometimes when we do that we lose sight of the bigger picture.

This is often the case in Western Medicine. By breaking down the structure of diseased cells into more and more minute parts, it often isolates these cells from the bigger picture of what's really going on in the entire body. It then tries to find a chemical that will have some bearing on this secluded group of diseased cells. The Chinese do the complete opposite, instead of just looking at this one illness in isolation in one part of the body, they will expand the picture and bring in every aspect of the body and all things affecting it from the environment into their view. They can from there see the bigger cause of the illness. Or see whatever weakness is in the body that has allowed the illness to start.

For example in Western Medicine, you might have a toothache in your mouth, heartburn in your stomach, irritable bowel syndrome in your intestines, acne on your face, stress and anger in your head and a burning sensation from your urine. In Western Medicine, everything will be reviewed as isolated problems without connections. You will be sent to a dentist for the toothache. A digestive specialist for the heartburn and irritable bowel syndrome. A skin specialist for the acne. A psychiatrist for the stress and anger issues. And a urinary specialist for the burning urine. In Chinese Medicine you will see just one doctor. The same Chinese medical practitioner will build up a big pattern from all those symptoms and see what links them together. In this simple case, heat is the common denominator for them all, (you will see how to come to this conclusion later on in the book). The doctor may give you a herbal formula to clear general heat with extra herbs added to cool more localised areas. When you start to clear away the overall heat you will see a reduction in all of the above symptoms. They will eventually all fade away.

Herbs are seen in Chinese Medicine as stronger more potent versions of foods. They can give quick and powerful effects in treating illness. However you will see later that there are many simple foods we can buy in our local stores that are perhaps a little slower to work but are often very effective in treating illnesses.

Through questioning and examining, the Chinese doctor will gather many symptoms from all parts of mind and body to produce the real causes of illness. No single symptom is ever viewed in isolation. We must look at the big picture to see what created it.

Sometimes when we are concentrating on the small details we lose sight of the obvious that is right in front of our eyes. This can be seen when we look at some Western diagnostic methods, such as microscopes and blood tests. They are very useful for seeing and measuring diseased cells in the body. But they are not so good at determining the strength in an individual, and therefore that individuals strength to combat germs, recuperate from and fight illness. For example, a ninety year old and a twenty year old may both have had a blood test that shows them to be disease free. However, it's very likely that the twenty year old is much stronger and in better health than the ninety year old. This will not be shown through medical tests and instruments. But is easily seen by the eyes.

The big picture is also very important in all other aspects of our health. Not just in the treatment and causes of illness but also in the prevention of illness and creation of good health. In order to create excellent health we need to focus on all areas of our lives and environments. These areas include mind, emotions, spirit, soul, diet, exercise, sex, climate, sleep, work and so on. You cannot just have a perfect diet or exercise regimen and ignore the rest. Although some may have bigger impacts on you, all are fundamentally important for health and happiness of the whole being.

Chapter Six - Qi.

Qi is the Chinese name for the energy involved in all creation and existence. It quite simply moves, creates, transforms, maintains, activates and holds in place everything the human being and the universe is made of. It is the energetic life force of all existence. Every living thing throughout nature needs energy. Plants need the sun's energy to grow. They create more leaves in summer to pull more energy into them. Even eggs need chickens to sit on them, warm them and put energy into them, making them grow and hatch.

In simple terms, you can think of energy in the human body in the same way as you think of energy in batteries or power from electricity. When we put batteries or electricity into a machine it brings it to life. It animates it, it powers it up to function in whatever way it is intended to. However, if those batteries start to run out then problems occur. If you had a torch with failing batteries, the light would start to dim. Without sufficient power any machine will falter or not even work at all. The body is exactly the same, the weaker the energy, the more problems and ill health it will have. Organs will weaken and be unable to create or move substances or perform their necessary functions. This will of course lead to illness in some form or another. Absolutely everything you do is dependant on energy. You cannot perform a single action without it. Every movement and even every thought and emotion is dependant on it, to give it life.

By simply increasing overall energy in the body you will find that you can cure many problems. Every organ and cell in the body will be more powered up, will work better, be more productive, more healthy, more able to get rid of phlegm and toxins and so forth. The mind too, will have more ability to focus and control events in the body. By even further increasing energy, you will find the body brimming with life. Your health will become radiant and everything will run at their peak levels. You will find many techniques in this book which are solely regarding the building and maintaining of maximum levels of energy in the body.

So how does all this fit in with modern science ? Well Western Medicine sticks to the old Newtonian view of physics. However, things have moved considerably forward since then. With Albert Einstein came the atom and the beginnings of Quantum Physics. In Quantum Physics everything is seen as energy. As Einstein said "mass is merely another form of energy". All matter and physical objects, including us, are seen at their smallest levels as particles of energy. To most people when they first hear about this it seems absurd. For they can touch everything around them and sure enough it appears to be solid. But when you start to think of it in a different way you can easily see how energy can create seemingly physical objects. For starters, if you were to touch electricity (not advisable !) or be hit by lightning (again something you really want to avoid !), its energy will physically knock you back.

Atoms themselves are composed of a nucleus and charged electrons which fly around it. Between these two we have empty space. So much empty space that if a nucleus was a baseball in a baseball park, you would have to go outside the park before you would meet any electrons. In essence we are made of small electrical charges and mostly empty space! The electrons are flying around the nucleus so fast that it gives the illusion of a solid. To understand this you could imagine a fan with lots of empty spaces between the blades. When you switch it on and the blades are moving very quickly, it appears to form a solid. Or even tie a rope to a bucket and spin it really fast. No matter where you try to touch in the spinning circle it appears to be solid.

Every atom is radiating at a unique energy pattern and level of vibration. Sometimes atoms will lose their electrons. The flow of these charged electrons through the body generates electricity. Giving us the power to perform and animate our existence. Oddly most of Western Medicine ignores what quantum physics states and has stayed only at the materialistic level of Newton's principles. I have always found it interesting that one branch of Western science clearly ignores another and yet still claims to be scientific. The Newtonian style science of Western Medicine has been out of date with physicists for more than eighty years now. Televisions, computers, rockets, mobiles and lasers have all developed from the Quantum revolution. The atom bomb and nuclear weapons are also part of its history. Since Western Medicine has invested heavily in the use of chemical drugs, it seems very resistant to stray from this path. Perhaps if drug companies find a way to bottle and sell energy then we will very quickly be told of an astonishing new energy science and medical breakthrough that they have discovered.

Fortunately for us, we have many methods already in Chinese Medicine to build our energy. And most of them are absolutely free. Energy can be formed in many ways in the body. The Chinese character symbol for Qi gives us an indicator of where energy can come from. When you break down the symbol it refers to air and rice (food). Two major contributors to the energy in our bodies. It can also be created from the sun, from heat, from hormones and chemicals, from exercise and friction and even from our mind and spirit. Of course once you have a good level of energy in the body, you also need to be aware of all the things that can rapidly start to deplete it. Preservation of energy then becomes a vital focus. All these methods will be fully explained and discussed in later chapters.

Chapter Seven - The Art Of Balance.

Quite often in the East you will hear of the terms Yin and Yang. Taken literally, Yin means the dark side of the mountain and Yang means the bright side of the mountain. They represent the seemingly opposite states of life which interflow and eventually act to rebalance each other.

In practical terms, for example, after a long hot summer which dries out the earth and consumes its nutrients, we need a cool wet winter to nourish the land and bring it back into a healthy state of balance for the next yearly cycle. In man, for example, after being active all day, the body needs to rest at night, to recuperate and restore itself for a fresh start the next day. In nature after one state reaches its peak it generally starts to create the other. Night turns to day, heat turns to cold. Even molten lava eventually cools into hard cold stone. Everything ebbs and flows backwards and forwards in a state of constant change and mutual support.

In the body it is the same. We can swing from one set of conditions into another. However if we stay too long in any extreme state we can start to damage ourselves. To stay healthy we need to keep everything in the middle, reasonably balanced. If we were to do something that pushes away from this state of balance then we often become ill. For example, coffee, alcohol and spices all tend to create heat in the body. In wintertime when we are cold if we consume some of these we will heat up. This protects our bodies from the cold and brings them into a safe middle ground where everything is functioning the way it was intended to. These foods will actually help us, because too much cold would slow down our bodies and weaken them. However if it becomes quite hot in summer and we still consume these heating foods then we will find we begin to over heat on the inside. As the heat intensifies, it burns up the nutrients in the body and can start to badly damage cells leading to disease. Even too much sun in summertime often shows this as its intense heat can dry out and damage our skin, destroying cells and burning away nutrients.

To stay healthy we need to remain in the middle ground. Any extreme condition created in the body often causes ill health. Extremes can come from heat, cold, dryness or dampness and so on. They can be too much or too little of a substance or even the under or over functioning of organs.

Later we will discuss how to spot key signs of the body starting to go out of balance. If you can catch these signs in their early stages, then you can quite easily reverse them, remain healthy and avoid any ills they would most likely lead to. You will be shown many ways to alter states in the body throughout the book. A very simple and easy way is through our everyday foods. In the previous example of heat in summertime, you could alter this state by avoiding those heating foods and by introducing foods that create cold in our systems. In practical terms, once you have figured out what's gone wrong, you simply need to do the opposite. Too much cold, then heat things up. Too much stagnation, then get things moving. Too toxic, then flush the body clean. And so forth.

Throughout your life you will find your body constantly changes. As you age and naturally slow down, your body will need to be readjusted. If you are working or exercising too much or too little, your background life needs to be changed. If you become stressed or emotional, changes in the background can again offset this. In the winter cold, you instinctively are aware to put on extra clothes, perhaps a warm coat, hat and scarf. In summer heat, you know to do the opposite, such as a t-shirt and a pair of shorts. With the right knowledge, you can learn how to balance the rest of your life as easily as you do your clothing for the weather. Through this, you will find you can successfully manage your body and avoid the states and conditions that will lead to and cause most sicknesses.

Chapter Eight   -   We Are All Still Part Of Nature.

The human being, in its current form Homo Sapiens, has according to most historians been on this planet for about the last 80,000 to 140,000 years. Our bodies have been in roughly the same form all this time. Because of this they have evolved in a certain fashion and we are stuck in those ways. We cannot break free from them in the space of 10, 20, 50 or even a 100 years. In past times when it became bright, people would get up, hunt, gather foods, and then eat them. When it got dark they would go off to bed and sleep. There was not much else they could do. Obviously they could not stay up and watch television, do shift work, eat meals or anything else throughout the night.

Because of our slow evolution, we are stuck with an internal biological clock that dictates when our bodies and its organs are functioning at their peaks for different tasks. For example, from morning to lunch, the energy in our digestive systems is at its most powerful. And at night, for about four hours after 10 to 11 pm, our bodies will emit growth hormones to repair, replace and rebuild cells.

Our bodies too are used to breaking down unprocessed, unrefined simpler more natural foods. They are not structured to deal with many of the additives and preservatives now found in our food supply. Our physical systems are not built to cope with life in a 24 hour society, nor are our brains designed to process the vast amount of information we are now being exposed to in our media and technology driven culture. Technology has very definitely well out paced us.

Science has provided us with many fantastic improvements and comforts in our lives but we must never forget that our bodies are part of nature and the more we move out of our natural rhythms the more sick we tend to become. Sometimes common sense is more beneficial to our lives than scientific fact. For example, we all know the earth undeniably revolves around the sun. This is an indisputable fact. However, the common observation of the sun moving over our heads and across the earth from morning to night, giving it the appearance of revolving around the earth, has many more practical implications for the human being. It dictates our sleep, our work, our meal times and even times for socializing. Sometimes common sense, practical and natural approaches are much more influential, important and relevant to our everyday lives than technical science is.

Chinese medical science tends to try to fit in with more natural laws and observations. It is more concerned with functioning and practical responses than with minute structures of cells. Most often as long as we are making the right changes on the bigger level, then all the smaller parts which make it up will automatically change right along with this bigger process. Chinese Medicine sees nature as having superior knowledge in its own design and its design of the human being. It therefore tries to assist and guide people back into a natural state allowing their own bodies to perform the complex healing at microscopic levels. The body created itself in the first place. And when it is given the opportunity and right circumstances provided by Chinese Medicine and right living, then it truly knows best how to rebuild and heal itself.

Chapter Nine - The Organ System And Vital Substances.

The main organ systems in Chinese Medicine revolve around the heart, the liver, the kidneys, the lungs and the digestive organs. These will all be explained in more detail as it becomes necessary. For the moment, all we need to know is that the organs in Chinese Medicine represent entire systems in the body. Every aspect that can come from an organ is put into its system. This includes all physical, emotional, mental, energetic and even spiritual aspects. For example, cold feet and broken weak finger nails can be related to the livers inability to regulate and release the blood it stores. Therefore these symptoms would all be combined into the system relating to the liver. Whereas in Western Medicine when they speak of the liver, they tend to solely focus on the physical organ. Chinese Medicine is more interested in the bigger picture, the functioning of the organs and their influence throughout the entire body. It also examines how they interrelate to each other and to the bodily substances and the environment.

The Vital Substances Of The Body.

Along with energy in our bodies, for this book we will need to know about a few other substances which have a very important impact on our systems. The ones we will discuss here are blood, essence and spirit.

Blood in Chinese Medicine is seen to have moistening, nourishing and cooling properties. It partners with energy to provide all the basic essentials for everyday living. As it enters through the lungs it combines with energy from the air and the two are pumped around the body to feed and support cells, organs, mind and all other parts. In healthy abundance they can even support our emotional and spiritual well being.

Blood and energy tend to balance the temperature of the body. Energy by its nature is hot. The more active it gets the hotter it gets. We can see this very clearly in nature, the sun gives us incredible amounts of energy and with it comes heat. When you exercise and create energy through movement you become hotter. With electricity, if you were unfortunate enough to get a shock, you would also receive burns from it.

As molecules are heated they start to vibrate more intensely. This movement generates more and more heat. Eventually the molecules will separate, take up more space as they bounce and smash against each other and turn themselves into a gas. As they cool they do the opposite. The molecules and atoms will move slower and slower, and start to condense and combine. They will begin to form solids. The more slow they get the more dense and heavy they appear to be.

In nature we generally see that the more heavy and dense an object appears to be the more cold it seems to our touch. Minerals like stones and steel quite simply feel cold when we touch them. When something feels cold it is taking energy from us. When something feels hot it is giving us energy. For example, if we stand in the hot sun our bodies are absorbing energy. If we were to stand outside in the cold and snow our bodies would lose energy.

Blood is composed of dense components from our food such as proteins and minerals. The cold that comes from these acts like a balance to the heat that comes from our energy, keeping our temperature at reasonable levels in the body. When the body repeatedly loses this balance between heating energy and cooling blood, then many illnesses are often formed.

Spirit in Chinese medicine is a combination of our mind and soul. It runs our system and gives direction, purpose and meaning to our lives. When we are in good spirits, our energies and bodies thrive. When we become sad, low or feel down, everything runs more slowly and less effectively. This eventually stagnates fluids and organs, and then weakens and breaks parts in our bodies leading to actual physical diseases.

Finally we have essence or to give it its proper Chinese name, Jing. Jing in Western terms would mainly be seen as hormones, DNA, stem cells, sexual fluids and even brain marrow. It would be all the deepest essences of the human body. For reproduction, Jing creates the egg and sperm and controls and supports reproductive organs. In life it is the backbone of our health. It is responsible for the regeneration of all our cells. If we find ourselves in trouble and our energy and blood cannot fix our circumstances then Jing is released as powerful hormones such as cortisone and adrenalin to come to our aid. When we are born we inherit a certain amount of Jing from our parents. The harder we live our lives, the more quickly we will use that Jing up. And as it weakens and runs low, we will age more quickly and find it more difficult to heal and recover from stressful situations that life often throws at us. Because of this, it is seen as essential in Chinese Medicine to preserve your Jing as much as possible if you wish to lead a long and healthy life.

Section Two - The Causes Of Illness.

Chapter Ten - Genes And Germs.

Before we look at the Chinese causes of disease, we must look at two aspects of Western Medicine which they project as the cause of many diseases. These are genes and germs.

Genes.

Genes are blueprints of how cells should perform. They can contain predisposing elements which may lead to disease. When scientists initially discovered them, they believed whatever genes you inherited at birth would manifest your future health or illness. Nowadays thanks to epigenetics we are starting to see a very different picture. Epigenetics show how the environment is really controlling our genes. The environment that we are in can switch them on or off. Anything that you do which weakens or aggravates your body, can turn on the DNA inside your cells to produce disease.

The big picture here, is that for most of us, you have to still lead an unhealthy lifestyle to become sick. There is a small percentage of people, about two percent, who scientists suggest have certain unavoidable traits in their genetic make up. But for most of us it comes down to what we all knew before. If we smoke, if we eat the wrong foods, if we don't learn how to deal with stress and so forth, then we are likely to become ill. If we do live healthy lives, we are far less likely to suffer.

Many studies have shown that after a period of time, immigrants to the US who come from a healthy gene pool such as Japan, still become unhealthy and get the same incidence of disease as regular US citizens, regardless of the good genetic make up they have. The Japanese are credited to have the longest life span in the world, they suffer from considerably lower levels of cancer, heart disease and other ills than those in the US, so are considered to have better genes than them. However, when they live in the US and adopt their lifestyle they get just as sick as everyone else there.

We can also look at obesity to see that genes are not responsible for it. The obesity epidemic has only really come into existence in the last ten to twenty years. As I said earlier, we have been on the planet in this form for over 80,000 years. So our genes certainly haven't suddenly changed in this generation to make most of us overweight. We are becoming overweight from eating too much of the wrong types of foods. From the many indigestible chemicals and substances that now infiltrate them and our environment. Not from our genes. The current children being born to overweight adults will most likely inherit these altered genes but the vast majority of adults alive today certainly did not.

Occasionally you will come across an adult who has weak digestive genes that they were born with. I was one of them. I was born weighing about ten pounds, quite a big baby for that time. I grew up fat as a toddler and child. I ate roughly the same foods as my brother, but whereas he remained a normal weight I was much heavier. Up until the age of thirteen, when I started exercising vigorously every day, I was considerably overweight. I was the fattest kid in my class and indeed in most of the school for many, many years. After learning Chinese Medicine I was able to use their techniques to alter and enhance my digestive system and whereas most adults in Ireland are now overweight and obese, I maintain a normal healthy weight. So even if you are born with weak genes, it certainly does not mean that you are stuck with them. What you do in your lifestyle after you are born is far more important and has far more of an impact than what you have inherited.

A study by Chris Murgatroyd and others at the Max Planck Institute Of Psychiatry, reported in the journal Nature Neuroscience, found that exposure to early life trauma in mice, changed their DNA. Stress hormones released in them, actually tweaked the DNA codes of a set of genes in these mice. Leaving them more susceptible to long term behavioural problems.

Research by scientists at the Patiala University in India, suggested that background exposure to pesticides has altered and damaged the DNA of people in farming communities, which has led to higher rates of cancer amongst them.

A study by Dean Ornish and colleagues at the Preventive Medicine Research Institute and the University Of California, published in the Proceedings Of The National Academy of Sciences, found that good nutrition, emotional support, moderate exercise and stress management, changed the expression of the genes in over 500 men with prostate cancer, within a three month period. With these good healthy lifestyle changes, it was found that many disease promoting genes were down regulated or turned off and many protective disease preventing genes had been up regulated and turned on in these men.

Germs.

Western Medicine often looks for bacteria and viruses to be the sole sources of human illnesses. This way of thinking originated way back in the 1800's from Louis Pasteur who is recognised as the father of The Germ Theory. The Germ Theory states that when we are exposed to bacteria and viruses they make us sick. Since then Western Medicine has spent vast amounts of time and money trying to create drugs that will kill these bacteria and viruses. Unfortunately many of these same drugs often weaken the rest of us too, often depleting our energy and resources, and even weakening our bodies natural defence, our immune system.

The Chinese approach is quite different. They would respect that germs can certainly make you ill, but whether you get sick or not has more to do with the strength and power of certain elements in your body. In particular your energy system. If you have abundant energy and your immune system is fully powered, then it can easily produce white cells, the bodies defenders. If this is the case, it is difficult even when exposed to germs to become sick. You will learn much more about strengthening your body to this level later on in the book.

It's quite clear to see that there is much more to the causes of illness than just germs. Otherwise everyone exposed to an illness would develop it and this is clearly not the case. Doctors, nurses and health care workers are constantly around patients with infections all the time, yet most of the time they don't get anything. They simply don't become sick from this exposure. Everybody usually knows someone in their circle who never seems to get colds or flu during winter but must also have been exposed regularly to these bugs. In fact we are constantly surrounded by thousands and thousands of germs on a daily basis. They are everywhere, our bathrooms, kitchens, computers, beds and nearly all other places. Even our cars have registered to have more than 15,000 different types of bugs in them. So it is more than obvious that germs are only one side of the equation and for that matter the smaller side.

Chapter Eleven - The Causes Of Illness.

The next section of chapters are probably the most difficult to grasp in the entire book. Many of the concepts in this part will be quite new for the Western way of thinking. If you initially find some of these ideas confusing then don't worry. By the time you have read the rest of the book, everything will come together and start to make sense. After you get through this section, you will find that the rest of the chapters are much more self contained and are therefore easier for Western minds to follow. A lot of the methods described later are stand alone techniques which don't require you to have an in depth knowledge of Chinese Medicine in order to make them work. However, the more theories you understand and the more you can put them into practice, the better and healthier you will be able to make your life. So I have included extra knowledge in this section. But remember not to fret, as you don't need to understand or remember all of it to derive great benefit from this book.

The Causes Of Illness.

There are many different actions that can lead to problems and illnesses in the body. Ailments can come from a sudden or severe impact on a system that is not in strong health. This could be an attack from a virus or an intense fright or shock.

Or they can come from a build up of repeated actions of an inappropriate behaviour. Such as constantly eating the wrong foods, always over working or being continuously stressed for long periods of time.

They can come from a lack of something. Such as a lack of nutrients from good quality food, a lack of oxygen from poor breathing methods or even from a lack of love.

They can also come from inheriting a poor constitution or in Western terms, bad or weak genetic codes. If our parents were unhealthy or there was poor health or stress during pregnancy, then this is often passed onto the child, creating imbalance in them from the moment they are born. These are just some of the conditions that can cause illness but no matter where it originates from, its effect is to always throw the body out of alignment.

Once you know how to read the signs of a body that has become unbalanced, then if the person involved does not modify their lifestyle, you can quite often predict the future illnesses they could get and their outcomes. Illnesses like heart attacks, strokes and cancers don't just suddenly appear out of the blue. They are the climax of a steadily deepening progression of a bodily state that has become out of balance, probably many many years before.

For example, if someone constantly eats overly spicy hot and rich foods, they may initially get a stomach ache or heartburn. If they continue with the same diet, this may block up and overheat the stomach, leading to chronic heartburn. If the chronic heartburn is left untreated then the burning stomach acids may damage the cells in the lining of the oesophagus, the tube between the mouth and stomach. These damaged cells may eventually mutate and become cancerous. If a system in the body becomes out of balance and is left untreated, it may progress and develop over time into something far more serious. However, if it is treated and the condition is reversed and brought back into alignment, then the risk of serious illness greatly diminishes.

The external causative factors of disease, such as poor diet, unhealthy sleeping habits or stress, and how to avoid them will be discussed in detail in their appropriate chapters throughout the rest of the book. For the moment, in this section, we will concentrate our minds on the internal patterns in the body that they often create.

Firstly, a word of warning. This book is primarily designed to enhance your general health and teach you how to avoid illnesses. However, in this chapter we will discuss many actual diseases and problems. You will learn in future chapters how to address and resolve many of these issues through changes in your diet and lifestyle. If you are willing to make the right changes which alter the bigger pictures and also have some patience you will find lots of your problems will reduce in intensity and many may completely disappear. But the body can be very complex and while we will review the major patterns you can fall into, you will find that you can sometimes have one, two or even more patterns active in the same body at the same time. So if you are unsure and you think the patterns affecting you are too complex or if the illness is of a serious nature then contact a professional Chinese medical practitioner for help and guidance.

With a professional, be it Chinese or Western Medicine, make sure they are giving you plenty of time to explain your condition. How you most likely got sick. What you need to do to get better. How you can stay healthy and prevent reoccurrence of the illness. And even how you can improve your overall general health. If a doctor is unwilling to spend time with you and answer your questions, then you are better off finding another professional who will. Always be respectful and grateful to your practitioner, (a lot of us do work very hard to help you), but never be afraid to ask loads of questions and get good quality treatment from them.

Chapter Twelve - Patterns.

Once something has been sent out of balance, it starts to create a pattern inside of us. These patterns can create a chain of related symptoms that can affect many areas in the body. The simplest patterns are based around heat, cold, dryness, toxins, damp and phlegm. So if you are affected by a pattern of heat, then it may generate multiple symptoms of heat and damage from it throughout your system. Or a pattern of damp may create many symptoms relating to an excess of fluid in you.

In turn these patterns tend to create a big impact on our energy, blood, Jing essence and organs. They can also often combine and mix together to complicate things. Heat can combine with toxins or heat with dryness. And cold with dryness or cold with phlegm and damp.

With these patterns the easiest way to see the reactions they will cause in the body is to focus on what they do in nature. The way they behave outside of the body is also the way they behave inside of it.

Let's Start With Heat.

When we look at heat in nature we see it enlivens things. It energizes them. It gives them power and makes them run faster. In spring and summer, it brings animals out of hibernation and it grows flowers and plants. It warms and gives light and energy. However if heat becomes too excessive it can start to burn and dry. Plants will wither. The ground will become barren, hard and even start to crack.

In the body when we become too hot, internal parts speed up and become overactive. Our hearts may beat too fast. Our minds can become hyperactive and fill with anxiety. Our cells if they become too hot may start to mutate. Our nutrients may be burnt up, leading to an overall lack of nourishment in the body. This will cause a reduction in our energy, as part of its fuel source is burnt away.

Another feature of heat is expansion, when you heat fluids, molecules in them intensify activity, separate and take up more space to form gases. In the body this has massive implications causing inflammation and pressure. If you combine it with phlegm and toxins, they take up even more space in blood vessels and so forth in the body. The pressure can build up to such an extent to cause vessels to burst and rupture leading to serious damage. The other effect from swelling would be pain, as the pressure on nerve endings and the flow of energy increases and blocks up, pain will also follow.

Heat also causes things to rise. We can easily see this in nature through the simple process of rain. The sun's heat evaporates water, causing it to turn into a gas and rise up. As it cools, it condenses, becomes heavier and falls as rain. In the body, heat tends to rise up and cause lots of illnesses agitation and symptoms in the head.

Heat can often combine with dryness. Dryness, just as in nature, reduces fluids. This speeds up the process of withering things. Heat and dryness together can burn up precious cooling minerals, further upsetting the balance of hot and cold. And thus causing an escalation in damaging heat. Dryness can make things stiff and hard to move. As lubrication disappears things will become more grinding and will catch, tear and cause pain. Our blood and Jing levels can also be dried up and diminished. This will affect many parts of us, including our minds and spirits.

In the West, due to our rich diets, heat most commonly combines with toxins. In summertime if we leave food out in the open, it will quickly start to rot and putrefy. Bacteria loves damp and hot conditions. They feed and thrive in it. In nature you will always see insects gathering around stagnant murky pools and swamps in the heat. Just like flies and other insects are drawn to rotting, festering, decaying food, bacteria at a microscopic level also loves these conditions. The more hot and toxic your body is, the more perfect breeding grounds you have created for bacteria. Another thing you will notice with heat and toxins is that fluids become darker in colour and more odorous. Moist rotting food if left in hot and humid weather will brown in colour and become foul smelling. The more heat, the more activity, the more rotting will occur.

Next Up We Have Cold.

Cold flows hand in hand with lack of energy and lack of power. This leads to a general slow down and lack of activity in the body. In nature in winter, we see animals hibernate. They retreat, withdraw and try to hold on to their stores of energy through the cold months. Trees lose their leaves to preserve nutrients and energy. Most flowers and plants will disappear back towards the ground. As cold intensifies and depletes energy, even our car engines and their batteries can find it more difficult to charge up enough power to get themselves going.

Cold often tends to congeal and thicken substances. In winter, we will see condensation build up on cold glass mirrors and windows. We will see dew on the grass in the mornings. When it rains it will leave puddles and wet roads. Whereas in hot weather in the summer we get the opposite, things dry very quickly, even after a heavy rainfall.

In the body cold tends to do several things. It firstly steals energy, slowing down the organs and the mind. In extreme cold, hypothermia, everything starts to shut down. Even your mind loses its ability to think and concentrate. When things are not being processed they begin to pile up. Fluids and phlegm are created. As more and more substances, such as heavy minerals gather, this can lead to a further increase in cooling.

Cold also contracts, tightens, seizes and makes rigid. If you put your hand onto something cold, such as ice, you will feel it clench up. Internally, this can further impede functioning and cause more problems. Oddly this clenching can start to generate heat. As energy exists in everything, even in cold conditions, there is always still movement, be it ever so slow or slight. You will find this even in a dead body, where there is still a little energy helping to decompose it from one state into another. In our living bodies we have a huge amount of energy and as cold causes our muscles to tense, the body is still trying to push blood through these tissues and muscles. The vibration and activity of energy used to push the blood into these tight muscles starts to generate heat. If we are out in the cold sometimes we will get red noses and cheeks as extra energy causes heat as it pushes through these contracted blood vessels. In frost bite our tissues will actually burn and blacken. As hot energy battles against extreme cold, it ends up burning up its own tissues. If you freeze meat you won't get this effect. You will only get it in a living body which continues to pump energy into fingers and toes and other areas which can be affected by frostbite.

Another feature of cold is its ability to preserve. Whereas heat can dry or rot, wither and burn resources causing aging and putrefaction to speed up, cold does the opposite. It slows and preserves. We can see this very obviously by the use of our refrigerators to cool and preserve food.

Cold can also combine with dryness. Usually this comes from the weather in autumn and winter. Cold dry air and winds, can damage our lips, lungs and skin. It can start to drain fluids from our bodies.

However, cold more frequently combines with and can itself cause dampness and phlegm. When there is cold or a lack of warming heating energy, fluids are not processed and start to gather and block up our bodies. Causing swelling and impeding the free flow of movement through our systems.

Sources Of These Patterns.

Heat, cold and the other patterns can come from outside forces such as the weather and the seasons. Or even from work conditions, such as in air conditioning or in hot kitchens and so on. They can also manifest from more internally related conditions, such as consuming hot spices or cold ice cream and so forth. They can even come from heat or cold generated from emotional states such as anger and fear.

Another way to develop heat and cold is from a lack of their partner to balance the temperature on the inside. If you do not have enough heating energy then cold substances will predominate and you will become cold on the inside. Or the opposite can occur, for example, if you have not been eating enough vegetables, a very good source of heavy cooling minerals, then your ordinary correct levels of heating energy won't have a partner to cool them down and you will start to overheat on the inside.

Chapter Thirteen   -   Diagnosis.

In Western Medicine, diseases are always given unique and individual titles. In Chinese Medicine, instead of giving disease names to refer to illnesses, they give a descriptive picture of the state the illness is actually causing inside the body. We can look at two examples of lung disorders to see how this works.

Firstly if we look at asthma in Chinese Medicine, we find it is categorized in several different ways. We will discuss just two of these patterns. The first is known as the retention of phlegm and heat in the lungs. This may have come from having a very rich and hot diet, filled with phlegm and heat producing foods such as dairy, alcohol and sweets. The heat from the alcohol tends to cook, congeal and thicken the phlegm in the lungs turning it into a yellowy green mucus. This simply blocks up the passageways in the lungs, making it very difficult to breathe properly.

The second pattern involves the opposite. You may find it in someone who is often cold and tired. Their energy system is so weak that they have not enough to power up their lungs to properly oxygenate their bodies. You will find the cold air steals more energy from them in winter and often weakens them further. So in this case, you have two completely different patterns which are capable of creating the same disease. One is based on having an excess of heat and toxins in the lungs. Whereas the other has cold and a lack of energy in them. To be successfully cured, they both must be treated in completely different ways.

Another example that could affect the lungs would be a simple cough. One cough may come from heat and dryness on the inside. Another may come from cold and phlegm. Obviously, you will again need to match up the symptoms with the medicine to cure the cough. If you were to give stimulating heating medication to a cold phlegm cough. It would create energy and heat, and dry up and disperse the phlegm to get rid of it. However, if you gave those same heating herbs to a hot dry cough, you would dry things up even more and make it far worse. To properly diagnose and effectively treat a condition, you always need to build up the picture to see what's really happening in the affected organs. After that you simply do the opposite to bring the body back into alignment and balance. As the big picture changes, all the tiny ones are brought back into proper condition and functioning as well.

A word of caution. I have tried to keep this book as simple as possible to read, understand and to use in everyday living. Therefore I have purposely avoided putting the numerous over complex patterns and scenarios that exist in Chinese Medicine into this book. It would take many years of study to understand them all. I personally spent eleven academic years of my life studying all four branches of Chinese Medicine, Acupuncture, Tuina Medical Massage, Chinese Herbal Medicines and Medical Qi Gong. That's a huge amount of hours of intensive work. On top of that, I have learnt so much from years of practice, dealing with patients with every type of imaginable pathologies. So it's far beyond the scope of this book to fit all my knowledge or the vast knowledge of Eastern Medicine into it. However, what you do have, is a very useful and accessible, simplified guide. That should help you alleviate many illnesses and weaknesses from your life. And help you strengthen your body, mind and spirit to their maximum potential. But beware that if you are trying to treat illnesses, there are many complex patterns that can appear in the body. So if you are in any doubt, always contact a professional experienced practitioner for guidance and help.

An example of how complex patterns can sometimes develop can be seen in the following case. In this one, hot and cold patterns exist in the body at the same time. This can often be seen in people in the West who push themselves too hard, through work or even through too many late nights and partying too hard. In this case their most important organs for immediate survival, the heart and the liver, start to steal energy from the digestion and the kidneys, which are more vital for keeping us going long term. As the heart and liver speed up, to get through whatever workload they need to, they will usually start to overheat. Whereas the digestion and kidneys, as their energy is drawn away to the heart and liver, will start to cool down. This creates two patterns at the same time in the one body. Heat and over activity is above and cold and weakness is below.

Also sometimes organs may themselves be overheating, but will cause cold symptoms elsewhere in the body. The most common example of this, is provided by the liver. If it is working too hard, it can overheat and tire itself out. One of its functions is to store and regulate blood flow and glucose energy stores in the body. If it fails at this it can hold onto blood and not release it into circulation. If the heart has less blood to pump to the extremities, the hands and feet, then they will start to become cool and cold. This happens because they do not have enough turnover of blood with hot energy in it passing through them.

How Chinese Medicine Diagnoses A Condition.

It behaves like a detective. It starts with the local problem and then moves onto the other patterns in the body, gathering as much information and evidence from the disease and overall states as it can. Then it just joins the dots together to resolve the puzzle and reveal the big picture. In reality if you had ten symptoms, the majority of them will clearly point to the weakest underlying condition. But beware there are always one or two misleading symptoms that may point to other things. These are usually localised incidents. They are minor and in the background and are not the pressing issues that need to be addressed and resolved. They are like a hot liver causing cold hands, as discussed earlier.

In the next section, I have broken down the main patterns into the actual symptoms they may cause in the body. You can check any symptoms against them to reveal which pattern or patterns may be affecting you according to Chinese Medicine. If you suffer from a heat pattern you will not get all the symptoms you see in the heat section. You may only get a few. These will just be the ones that are relevant to your inherited genetic make up or the ones related to an inappropriate behaviour that is causing your illness. For example as heat builds up in the head and creates pressure, one person may get a migraine, another a nose bleed, another a racing anxious mind. And unfortunately for some, they might even get a combination of all three.

Sometimes you find people who fit mainly into hot patterns or others mainly into cold ones. If however, you end up in the category of people who have some overheated organs and some cool energy deficient ones, then this is more complicated and less straightforward to deal with. But if you follow the advice in later chapters, avoiding that which could be pressurising organs and causing them to overheat, while at the same time practising the methods that generate good clean energy in your body, then over time, your system should rectify and rebalance itself in a more middle healthy position. From there, if there is any illness or weakness left, it should be far easier to correct.

Chapter Fourteen - Illnesses And Symptoms Relating To Heat In The Body.

This chapter will list common symptoms relating to individual body parts in regard to heat, heat with phlegm and toxins, and heat with dryness.

We will briefly recap on heat before we begin. In general it makes things move faster, burns up nutrients, agitates and causes swelling and inflammation.

When combined with dryness, it severely attacks nutrients, oils, fluids and minerals. It seizes and tightens the body.

When combined with phlegm and toxins, it increases pressure. It blocks up processes. It starts to rot and destroy cells. And it provides a breeding ground for bacteria.

With heat, signs and symptoms tend to be bolder and more exaggerated. Pains will have more pressure, so they will usually be more intense, stabbing and throbbing. Skin, if affected, will generally be more dry, red, itchy, sensitive and raw. If toxins are present, it will have oozing or yellow pus filled blemishes. Urine will most likely be scanty and yellow, with perhaps a foul odour. Usually the bowel movement will be hot and dry producing constipation or wet, loose and odorous. The breath and body odour may also be strong smelling. The mood will be aggravated by heat and pressure causing irritability, frustration, anger, anxiety and racing in the mind. Often there can be heartburn if there is excessive heat in the stomach. Or headaches, tinnitus or blood shot eyes if there is heat and pressure in the head. The more heat that is present, the bigger these symptoms will appear.

Below is a list of possible symptoms that may be related to an overheated system. We will start at the top of the head and work our way right down to the feet. Listing all the symptoms that may possibly occur in each part along the way.

Do remember that these symptoms may be caused by other patterns. Just like we discussed earlier with asthma. So we are not looking at these symptoms in isolation but as part of a bigger picture, of a pattern of overall heat.

Starting At The Top.

Thumping migraine headaches - Particularly at the sides of the head and at the temples. This is caused by heat swelling the tissues and blood inside the brain. As your brain is encased in a skull, there is little space available for it to swell. So every time the heart pushes blood out into the body, the pressure gets too much inside the skull and nerve endings are squashed. Resulting in a thumping pain.

Tinnitus - Loud ringing in the ears is caused by heat agitating and inflaming the ear. Softer ringing is usually caused by a lack of cooling minerals in the ear. So there is not enough present to offset the heat from the energy and things begin to overheat in the ear.

Ear ache - Too much hot blood swells the blood vessels in the inner ear causing pressure and pain. It may be accompanied by dry skin or redness on the outer ear. Toxins and bacteria may also build up causing more pressure and pain.

Red face - Is caused by heat expanding the tiny blood vessels supplying the face.

Nose Bleeds - Hot blood expands and bursts blood vessels in the nose. This is usually quite forceful bleeding. There is too much pressure in the blood vessels, so the blood gushes out.

Racing or anxious mind - The heat is usually in the brain and the heart. It disturbs blood circulation through the brain, distressing it. The heat speeds and over activates the brain. Also blood and its nutrients can easily be burnt up, producing poor quality blood. This deficient blood fails to nourish and support the mind.

Anger, frustration and irritability - The heat is in the brain and in the liver. Expanded and heated blood agitates the mind and builds up pressure in it. If it is extreme you may blow your top and explode with rage. Heat also burns away good nutrients used for food and fuel by the brain, and burns away minerals used to cool it. So the brain is less able to think clearly and calmly.

Dry, red, tired, gritty, or sticky eyes - Heat swells the blood vessels in the eyes, expands them and gives them the "blood shot" look. It is commonly seen after consuming heat producing alcohol. Dry, gritty and sticky eyes can come from heat drying and congealing fluids on the eyes.

Mucus affecting the nose and sinus - If it's heat related, the mucus will usually be yellow, green or darker colours. If it's hot and dry the nose will be stuffy and blocked.

Broken veins on nose - Commonly referred to as a "Brandy Nose". Heat has permanently swelled and burst tiny capillaries on the nose. This sometimes results from over consumption of alcohol, but can also be from too much spices, coffee, dark teas, sugars and fats. Or even from anger and stress.

Sticky mouth, bad breath or bad taste in the morning time - Is usually caused by heat and phlegm in the stomach. This produces rotting odours and foul tastes.

Bleeding gums - Heat causes blood vessels in the gums to expand and swell. When pressed on by toothbrush bristles, they will easily burst and bleed. This is just like the way a balloon with too much air blown in it can burst easily.

Dental abscesses and toothaches - Can be caused by heat from foods such as sugars, coffee, alcohol and rich foods. It can also come from heat caused by stress. Heat swells blood vessels in the gums, causing them to put pressure on the teeth and squashing nerve endings. If the mouth is not clean then toxins can build up, increase pressure and pain, start to rot and cause infections. Toothaches are usually resolved through the use of herbs and corrections in diet in Chinese Medicine. Dentistry is not generally recommended.

Dizziness - Heat can cause pressure in the brain. It can also burn away nutrients from our blood, which can weaken it and leave it unable to support and nourish the brain.

Mouth sores - Heat can cause inflamed, swollen, tender eruptions.

Stroke - Heat in the blood vessels in the brain causes them to expand. If the pressure becomes too great, one can rupture and bleed into the brain causing massive damage.

Twitches in eyelids - Heat causes pressure to build intensely in little blood vessels in eyelids. Eyelids may twitch when extra pressure comes from the heart pumping blood out through the body.

Dandruff - The heat burns up nutrients in the blood and the scalp, so it is not fed, nourished and moistened. Causing it to appear dry and flaky.

Thinning, dry or frizzy hair - If the blood is hot and deficient in minerals and nutrients, then hair follicles are not fed and the hair becomes thin and dry.

Wrinkles - Heat can often dry up the skin, and burn up nutrients and minerals in the blood that should be nourishing and moistening it. This causes it to age more quickly. This can often be seen in smokers, sun bathers and coffee drinkers.

Dry mouth and thirst - Heat has burned up cooling and moistening fluids, leaving the mouth dry and thirsty.

General feelings of heat - Hot people tend to want to turn off heaters and radiators. And wear less clothes than others around them, (unless those others are suffering from too much heat as well).They also might stick their feet outside bed covers and kick blankets off themselves at night and so on.

Poor Sleep - Heat in the mind or body causes it to remain too active. This can cause restless sleep, difficulty getting to sleep or trouble staying asleep.

Night sweats - Usually caused by overactive hormones, or from excessive stomach heat, or a body filled with toxins.

Hot Flushes - Usually caused by overactive hormones. And a lack of cooling minerals and heavy substances to offset the heat.

Rashes, psoriasis, eczema, acne - Blood should nourish, moisten and supply the skin with minerals to keep it cool, but if it has become overheated, blood will instead inflame and dry out the skin causing rashes. If it has become hot and toxic, blood will heat and inflame the skin and try to push these toxins out through the pores. Some toxins will get caught in the pores blocking them and causing acne, infections or oozing rashes.

Cholesterol - Heat, toxins and phlegm gather in blood vessels. This can lead to blockages throughout the body and pressure increases in areas like the heart and brain. It can also cause the heart to overwork as it has to push harder to circulate blood through all the thick heavy phlegm and fats around the body. This can cause it to wear out quicker.

Tight, sore and achy muscles - Blood should nourish, soften and relax muscles. If it does not, then the muscles will become stiff and tight.

Rapid heart beat, panic attacks, thumping in the chest - Heat has over activated the heart, speeding it up. It needs to be cooled and slowed down.

Dry cough - Particularly active in evenings and at night. Heat in the lungs has dried out lubricants that allow flexible movement through them. Usually the lungs need oils and cooling minerals to resolve this.

Arthritis, sore inflamed joints - Heat can dry oils from joints causing them to seize and stiffen. Heat and toxins can jam up and lodge in joints, blocking off access for good fresh nutrients to help keep them strong and causing bad sludge to lodge in them instead. This can lead to pain as nerve endings are pressed upon.

Angina and chest pain - Heat and toxins clog up the blood vessels in the chest, causing swelling and pressure on nerve endings.

Dry, brittle, cracked nails - Blood is hot and nutrient deficient and fails to build and nourish nails.

Heartburn - Caused by an excessive build up of heat and acids. These are normally used to break down food. But when they become trapped and stay too long or get too intense in the stomach, pressure can build up, forcing them up the food pipe, causing a fiery burning sensation.

Strong appetite - Intense heat burns up food and its nutrients in the stomach. The brain and body does not get fed and then sends out signals for more food.

Emaciated or thin with feelings of heat in the upper body - The metabolism and body are too hot on the inside. It is burning and eating itself up.

Overweight or obese - If the digestive tract becomes overwhelmed with heat and toxic phlegm and sludge, usually from fatty, greasy diets. The body may start to retain them as useless fats and cause you to become overweight.

Cough producing yellow or darker phlegm - If heat related, the heat will thicken and cook the white clear phlegm, turning it yellow, green or darker colours. And causing it to rot and provide breeding grounds for bugs and bacteria. It will also make it smell and taste foul.

Tiredness with feelings of heat - This produces an uneasy feeling of tiredness. A kind of restlessness and dead energy. You can still get up and do things but you will feel tired at the same time. Like someone who has taken lots of alcohol, coffee or stimulants. Because you are hot, you still have a certain amount of energy in your body, but in this case you have burnt away all your fuel reserves, that is your nutrients from food. This is just like someone pouring petrol on a fire that is running out of logs. You are now running on the fumes of your energy, with no proper reserves and foundations.

Body odours - Heat and toxins over cook fluids in the body creating unpleasant smells.

Skin infections - Heat, phlegm and toxins lay the breeding grounds for infections.

Low or mid back pain - Heat agitates the kidneys, swelling them and their surrounding tissues.

Constipation - Heat has dried up the inside of the intestines, making it very difficult for food to pass through.

Odorous bowel movements - Heat makes things go off. Even in nature we see this quite clearly. Dog excrement is really foul smelling if left out in the heat and humidity in summertime. It attracts flies and bugs. If your stools are foul smelling, it means that your intestines have become like a rotten cesspool on the inside. Odour from bowel movements is a very strong indicator of heat and toxins in the body. And can often be seen as a strong warning sign of looming serious future ailments.

Yellow or smelly urine - Urine should swing from pale yellow or clear to deeper yellows throughout the day. If it is always yellow or smelly, you have too much toxicity in your body. Urine can also be cloudy if overwhelmed by toxins.

Painful or burning urination - Heat and toxins agitate and inflame the lining of the bladder and the kidneys.

Painful periods - Heat and toxins cause swelling and pressure and block up the flow of blood. This can cause it to clot, press on nerve endings and cause pain.

Periods too early - If periods are constantly arriving before twenty eight days, then heat is usually speeding up and over activating the cycle.

Infertility - Toxins may obstruct movement. Heat may damage nutrients in blood and affect the quality supplied to the reproductive organs.

Vaginal discharges that are yellow or deeper in colour - Heat has cooked and congealed fluids and may provide a breeding ground for bacteria.

Restless legs and fidgeting - Heat is in the bloodstream causing it to over activate muscles. Quite often there is also a deficiency of cooling minerals present.

Spider veins - Hot blood swells and enlarges blood vessels causing noticeable thread or spider veins.

Varicose veins - Heat and damp swell and overwhelm the blood vessels in the legs, damaging its system for retaining and keeping blood in place. This causes blood to pool in veins. Usually there is also a component of weak energy here.

Swollen ankles in hot humid weather - Heat and damp gathering in the lower body.

Smelly feet - Heat and toxins are gathering in the feet. Heat causes things to go off quickly, rot and smell bad. If there are heavy toxins in your feet, they will continue to smell bad even if you wash them every day. You need to remove toxins internally to get rid of the odour. This condition is usually seen in people who are very toxic and is a dangerous warning sign of overall ill health.

Nail infections - Heat and heavy toxins gather in the toes. The heat cooks and rots the gooey toxins, turning them into breeding grounds for bacteria. Germs love damp and heat, so infections can quickly lodge themselves into the nails and begin to feast on the moist, decaying, rotting tissues.

Gout - Heat and toxins are building up in the joint of the ball of the foot. Bad poisons and heavy toxins often gather in the extremities, the hands and feet. Particularly in the feet, as they are furthest away from the powerful circulation that the heart provides, therefore they may become lodged there and can't easily be cleared away.

Tongue - Will usually be red in colour from heat. Will have a creamy yellow or deeper coloured coating if heat and phlegm are present. And will usually have tiny cracks and no coating if heat and dryness are involved.

Pulse - Heat will over activate the heart and speed the pulse up.

Inflammation - Diseases in Western Medicine ending in "itis" are usually related to heat and toxins causing swelling and expansion in them.

To Sum Things Up.

Foul odours, yellow, green and darker fluids and mucus, and general feelings of heat, swelling and pressure, are all usually good indicators that your insides have become hot, toxic and polluted. As these symptoms increase, your chances of getting more serious and dramatic illnesses also increase sharply.

Heat when not balanced can be damaging in the body and can deplete its resources. But heat and toxins are often a much more deadly mix and should be well avoided.

Sometimes people who are over heated can be lulled into a false sense of security. They will generally have more energy and get up and go than others. A sense of spring in their step and even often more enjoyment and excitement in their life. They will most likely get less colds or even none at all. And because of these reasons, they presume that they are healthier than most others. Unfortunately this is not the case. They are less likely to suffer from long drawn out conditions, like those endured by people with cold patterns. But are more susceptible to suffer sudden and catastrophic illnesses like cancers, strokes and serious heart attacks.

In nature a similar scenario presents itself. If you think of a hot tropical island, all seems to be like a paradise. However, as natural earthly pressures arises from all that heat, this build up generates a forceful, devastating, damaging event such as a hurricane, a tidal wave, an earthquake or even a volcanic eruption. So to stay healthy, be particularly careful to watch for signs to ensure your body is not overheating.

Chapter Fifteen - Illnesses And Symptoms Relating To Cold In The Body.

To recap on the characteristics of cold. It slows things and reduces energy and power. It impedes movement and can block things up. It congeals, thickens and creates fluids. As things become more damp, they become heavier and sink. It can cause things to swell with fluid. Or to contract, stiffen and tighten, often with pain. Pains caused by cold tend to be more dull, achy, dragging and drawn out.

So Let's Begin.

Tiredness - Cold steals your energy and slows you down. It also weakens your digestive system and lungs, which through breathing and digestion are two of the main contributors of energy in your body. Thus it can create a chain reaction leading to even more tiredness.

Colds and flu - Without energy, the immune system fails to have enough power to generate white defender cells when the body is under threat. Leaving you open and defenceless to colds and flu.

General feelings of cold - Cold people will find it hard to warm up. They will want to keep turning the heat up and will wear more clothes than others. At night they may use more blankets on their beds and pull covers tightly over themselves.

Weight gain and fluid retention - If your digestion and metabolism are slow and cold, you will gain weight and retain fluid easily. Liquids will start to gather and thicken in the body. If there is not enough energy for them to be transformed and used, they may end up blocking many parts of the body. Fresh or cold fluids will generally be clear or white in colour.

Dizziness - Phlegm can gather in the head blocking up the circulation of fresh blood, energy and oxygen. Also if your digestion has weakened it may fail to create blood properly. A lack of it and the oxygen it contains may cause you to become light headed.

Headaches - Dull lingering headaches can be caused by phlegm obstructing circulation and a lack of clear energy and fresh blood rising to the head.

Nose - Mucus if present, will be clear or white. It can be copious, congealed or blocked. It is caused by lack of energy to process and expel fluids.

Ear Aches - Fluids block up the inner ear leading to pressure, swelling and pain. External cold can also attack the ear causing it to contract and become painful.

Depression - If the digestion has become weak and underproductive, there may be a lack of energy created to spark up the mind. And a lack of blood to nourish the brain.

Worrying and over thinking - Phlegm can block up the mind. Causing thoughts to become stuck and repeat excessively. There is also a lack of energy to provide clear logical thinking.

Fearful and timid - If there is a lack of production of stimulant and strengthening hormones like testosterone, cortisone and adrenalin, then we may become fearful and nervous.

Lack of motivation - Is often caused by a decrease in stimulant hormones. There are no surging hormones in the body and no get up and go.

Poor concentration and memory - There is a lack of energy and blood to keep mental functioning, powered up and running at proper levels.

Blood - The production of blood can be very affected by cold, as its creator, the digestive system runs off of energy. And when cold and powerless, it is too weak to break down food and retrieve all the nutrients necessary to form healthy blood.

Pale or dull complexion - Caused by a lack of energy and blood to the face.

Numbness or pins and needles - Caused by lack of production of blood and deficient energy to move blood circulation. So blood sits, stagnates and begins to clot, pressing on nerve endings.

Palpitations and slow heartbeat - There is not enough energy for the heart to function at the right pace.

Breathlessness - There is inadequate power to keep lungs working effectively. Cold air can also cause them to contract, tighten and seize up.

Cough with white or clear phlegm - Fluids are not being forcefully expelled or dried up and instead they gather in the lungs congesting them. There can be copious amounts of phlegm or bubbly clear sputum.

Lower back ache - Unprocessed fluids are piling up in the kidneys and swelling them out, causing pressure inside them and on surrounding tissues and muscles.

Digestion - Digestion will be severely affected by lack of power to transform and process foods. Leading to indigestion, bloating, discomfort and loose or watery stools without any odour.

Urine - There may be large amounts of clear or pale yellow urine. The kidneys have not enough energy to filter bloods properly and remove toxins effectively. So they remain in the bloodstream and do not discolour the urine. The urine will not have any foul odour.

Periods - Can be heavy and painful as cold contracts and clots blood. The cycle itself can be slow and be over 28 days.

Bruising - The blood easily leaks from its vessels as there is not enough energy to form it properly and to keep it held in place.

Bleeding - Cold tends to cause blood to leak from vessels. These bleeds tend to be difficult and slow to stop. They don't gush but tend to drip instead.

Varicose veins - Blood pools in veins in legs, as there is not enough energy to keep the blood vessel retention system held in place and working properly.

Swollen ankles - The kidneys are not strong enough to process fluids properly. These end up gathering in the lower body causing the hips, knees and ankles to swell.

Arthritis - Cold can lodge in joints. This causes them to contract and slows down circulation through them. As fluids and nutrients pass through, deposits can build causing swelling and pain.

Cold, blue or purple hands and feet - Poor circulation from lack of energy causes reduced turnover of blood through the feet. However, cold hands and feet can commonly come about from an overheated liver, which fails to release enough blood and energy for the heart to pump down to the extremities, which in turn causes them to cool down.

Tongue - Fluids are being retained, so the tongue is usually flabby, swollen and may have teeth marks at the sides. It may also have a thick clear or white phlegm coating.

Pulse - Will usually be slow from lack of energy in the heart. If affected badly by cold then the pulse can contract, making it feel like a tight straight wire.

To Summarize Cold.

Generally diseases and illnesses that come from and are related to cold are usually more slow, chronic and drawn out conditions. With cold there is a slowing down of energy which can also lead to a slowing down in the brain and head, leading to a less stimulating, quieter and unexciting life. When there is a lack of energy even the eyes and ears may be affected. Eyes when functioning with less power will receive objects more dimly and less colourfully and ears will hear them less sharply.

Chapter Sixteen - Supreme Health.

At this stage it should be becoming clear, that in order to have a healthy body, mind and spirit, we should always strive to stay balanced and keep ourselves in the middle. Avoiding any extremes, not letting our systems become too hot, too cold, too damp or too dry.

In this way, you will keep all bodily functions running exactly as they are supposed to. They will have enough energy and power to carry out all their jobs effectively, and to keep your mind, bright, smart and happy. They will also have enough oils to lubricate all your parts. And nutrients to create more energy, nourish your cells, and be used in the rebuilding and regeneration of your physical body.

When the body has been brought into balance, it should be disease and ailment free. From here you can build on both sides, the nutrients and the energy, the Yin and the Yang. By doing this carefully and keeping levels balanced, you can build yourself up to supreme levels of health.

You can think of it like a fire that has been balanced with the right amount of logs and petrol to produce good effective flames, heat and light. Now that it is going properly, we can keep adding more logs and petrol as needed to build up the fire stronger and stronger.

The rest of the book is dedicated to teaching you and providing you with all the necessary information needed to bring you into balance. And from there, showing you what to do next to achieve the higher levels of supreme health.

Section Three - Food And Diet.

Chapter Seventeen - Introduction To Chinese Dietary Therapy.

Chinese Dietary Therapy is one of the great gems of Chinese Medicine. For thousands of years the Chinese have been gathering information on how herbs and foods digest and function inside the body. Through this observation, they have formed theories and principles that are clearly effective and correct. In comparison, it is not hard to see that Western nutritional advice is still in its infancy. For starters, it constantly seems to change its advice. Often completely reversing previous positions it has held. Its basics of proteins, carbohydrates and fats are too simple to give us good clear advice on what we need to consume to stay healthy. Even in relation to fats, it is only in recent history, the last ten years or so, that we have started to hear about omega oils and that fats have now been split into two categories. We have good healthy ones, usually plant oils, and bad ones, usually animal or man made fats.

After viewing diet the Chinese way, it is easy to see that Western dietary guidance has a lot to learn itself and falls far short in producing good practical advice for people. Instead, it tends often to contradict itself, leaving people confused and bewildered, not knowing what is and is not good for them. For example, one study might tell us that alcohol is good for you, and then in a conflicting study three months later, it may have been linked to cancer and we are told to avoid it as it will hasten our demise.

One of the issues here is an inability to see the big picture. The Western viewpoint again uses the approach of isolation and reduction. Reducing foods down to their bare building blocks. Disregarding their more obvious differences and characteristics. All vegetables are heaped in together. All fruits are heaped in together. Carbohydrates like potatoes, rice, pasta and wheat are basically given the same status and so forth.

The reasoning behind this, is that science sees them all at their smallest chemical levels, as coming from within its list of elements. As of 2008, there are 117 different elements in existence. Things like calcium, potassium, plutonium, hydrogen and magnesium. To some scientists, these make up life. The human body consists of about 25 different elements that create it. Yes, it is scientifically true that when we keep breaking foods down to their smallest chemical elements, we eventually end up seeing that many things are made of the same ones. It is also scientifically true that we can find all the same elements that could build an entire human being, right in our own back gardens. All the same elements are actually out there lying in the ground. But these taken in their original forms are useless. Unless the essential fundamentals of life and purpose are added to them, they remain mere chemicals. As great and as spell binding as science is, there are still missing ingredients in it. Intelligence, wisdom and soul are clearly missing at this lower more basic level. Everything in existence is clearly unique and has its own properties, actions and even purpose for its existence in this universe. Be it human beings or even fruit and vegetables. Everything has its own exclusive design and special qualities. It is a gross error just to view things as simple parts rather than seeing them as an individual identity created from the sum and workings of all these interrelated parts together.

When we study food, one of the very first things we should do, is look at our reactions to them. It is not hard to see massive differences when we view it from this angle. Clearly when we bite into a bitter lemon we get an incredibly different reaction than from biting down on a sweet banana. Yet in the West, they are both just classed as fruits. In Chinese Medicine, this is very different, later you will be able to see the vital difference between them.

However, it doesn't just stop there. You will also learn ways of being able to judge the differences between fruits of the exact same type. Yes, as strange as it sounds, one bunch of red grapes can be quite different in its actions and uses in the body to another bunch of red grapes. As you read on in the next chapters, all this will become really clear.

The Chinese view diet as absolutely essential to human health. They also believe that it is not just responsible for maintaining good health, but in many cases it can be used to successfully treat illnesses and restore health. This notion is often ignored in Western Medicine, for what I would believe to be financial reasons. If people can treat illnesses successfully through the use of diet, then the Western medical industry becomes less needed and may start to lose profits. So it remains in certain business interests to downplay the effectiveness of common foods.

It is only in relatively recent history that most medical universities are now teaching some sort of dietary course to their students. This is long overdue. The founding father of Western Medicine, Hippocrates, knew diet was essential right from the beginning. As he stated quite wisely "He who does not know food, how can he understand the diseases of man ?". Food contains a great arsenal of weaponry, against sickness, disease and ill health. We must learn how to use it and understand it correctly. If we don't we will continue to allow it to make us sick and unhealthy.

Just as I spoke of earlier, when we get used to thinking in one method and mental structure, we can often start to miss the most obvious. It is bizarre that Western science can at times produce incredible and great phenomena, yet at other times seems completely oblivious to simple truths and common sense. Hopefully in the future by opening our minds, by looking from the perspectives of the big pictures as well as the small ones, then scientific researchers can make many new and great discoveries beneficial to all human kind. We are about to find out about the bigger picture in terms of food, as we explore some very different viewpoints in the splendour and genius of Chinese Dietary Therapy.

Chapter Eighteen - The Five Flavours.

Chinese Medicine uses completely different approaches to understanding foods and their actions in the body. One of these methods is the Five Flavours. They are sweet, salty, spicy, bitter and sour. Each taste has a very different reaction in the body, producing very different results. Generally, in small amounts, they have a beneficial reaction. Whereas in large amounts, they can disturb it and throw it off course, even producing illnesses in it.

However, if your body is already off balance, you will need to take in extra amounts of a food type with characteristics that will nudge you back into the middle, where you can regain your health. For example, if the body becomes too toxic, you will need to take in more foods that detoxify until you become clean again on the inside. Or if it has become too dry, you need to take in more foods that will moisten and astringe, to lock fluids into you.

So let's start to examine how each flavour works and what effects it will produce in the body. Bear in mind, that these are general characteristics that work in most cases, but there is always an odd food that causes an exception and seems to do its own thing.

The Bitter Flavour.

When you put something bitter into your mouth, like a slice of lemon, it causes it to tighten up and squeeze. Your tongue will nearly try to push its way out of the back of your mouth. As this is happening, you will notice that your mouth waters. The fluid washes away the bitterness and your mouth is left feeling dry. The cells in your body don't like anything that tastes bitter. They close up against it. As they are clamping up, they are squeezing fluid out to push the bitterness away. They are treating it like a poison. Just like that old expression "a bitter poison". As the cells push out fluids they also push out fats and toxins as well. This gives them a good cleaning.

The action continues the whole way down the digestive tract, causing cells to push toxins away and eventually out of your body. Some of the flavour is also absorbed into your bloodstream and circulated around you. Any tissues and organs it reaches will again reject it, by tightening away from it, pushing fluids against it, and releasing toxins as well. The whole of the body can be cleaned by the ingestion of bitter fluids, foods and herbs.

Another benefit from bitter foods is that because they have helped push sticky, fatty toxins away from the cells and organs, they have made the movement through them much freer. Because of this, the cells and organs use up less energy while doing their jobs. As less energy is used, less heat is produced and the body starts to cool down. Therefore bitter tastes are used to cool the body and clean toxins and fluids from it.

Many antibiotics are probably related to bitter foods and herbs. They share similar characteristics to each other. They both purge and flush toxins and bacteria from the body. Their side effects are also similar. For example, the bitter taste is constantly producing fluid wherever it touches. Some bitter fluids are directed into the intestines and they end up awash with large amounts of fluid. The bowel movement then becomes looser. This is also a common side effect to be found with many types of antibiotics. Another similarity is that if you take too much bitter taste or too intense bitter taste for a long period of time, then you can start to feel weak and tired. As good energy, nutrients and blood can end up being drained out of your body along with the bad stuff. Many people often complain of feeling fatigued after being on antibiotics. So from a Chinese Medical perspective they seem closely related.

Even in our kitchens and around our houses we can see the effectiveness of bitter products. You will notice that many washing up liquids and cleaning products, particularly ones dealing with fats, grimes and grease, use bitter lemon, orange, grapefruit, or lime in them. You can try a simple experiment to see its effects. If you get a greasy pan and put water onto it, it won't do much. If you wipe it about, you will make a sludge at best. But if you squeeze lemon juice onto it, you will start to see the fats break up. If you wipe this, the fats will easily start to remove themselves from the pan.

The natural fat buster and detoxifier in your body is bile. It's produced in the liver and the gallbladder. Chinese doctors sometimes in the past used animal biles as treatments. Can you guess what flavour it is ? That's right, it is bitter. Hence the old expression "as bitter as bile".

However, be careful when you are detoxifying or even trying to lose weight. If you try to drink stacks of intensely bitter flavoured lemon juice everyday to detoxify faster, you may end up over tightening your body, which will strangle some of the smooth movement on the inside, as the bitterness gets trapped in some places. This can damage circulation and badly affect the functioning of organs. As your cells violently contract against the extreme bitter lemon flavour, you will also end up stripping away the oils, nutrients, vitamins, minerals and energy that is keeping you healthy. So it is best to avoid consuming extreme bitter tastes. Unless you have something nasty you want rid of, like bacteria or a virus.

Also be careful combining bitter fruit and juices with nutritious food. In the West, they claim fruit is digested quicker than other foods. What is actually happening, is your stomach just like your mouth and everywhere else, is trying to push away that bitterness and quickly forces it out of itself. This can have the effect of flushing nutritious food, which has been combined with juices away before it has been sufficiently broken down. When this happens you may be unable to fully absorb its nutrients and the food is wasted. The exception is green tea, although it is bitter, it is too mild in its nature and is therefore fine and usually helpful to combine with any type of food.

The general rule for using the bitter flavour is to use plenty of it when you are in a hot and toxic state. Consume lots of green tea. Lots of juices like pomegranate, berries and grapes, up to about a litre a day. And if there are signs of active bacteria and infections, have watered down weakened lemon, lime or grapefruit juice for a while to help deal with them. One should also obviously stop taking in foods that are toxic and phlegm creating as well, as they are encouraging the growth of viruses and bacteria.

When we are balanced, we can have lots of weak bitter flavours, such as green tea or watered down juices. We should also have a glass or two daily of the more medium bitter tastes like pomegranate, berries and grapes. Intense flavours like lemon and grapefruit should be taken infrequently, perhaps once a week or even once every few weeks.

A century ago, there would have been less need to detoxify our bodies. But modern levels of pollution in our air, environment, water and food now means we have to constantly consume more of these natural cleansers to stay healthy. A government report in the UK in 2008 found that over 30 percent of our foods now contains traces of pesticides and chemicals. But don't worry, in my experience, once the body is reasonably clean and phlegm free, it can quite successfully, with a little help from our bitter fruits, juices and teas, eject any pollutants that may cause it harm.

When we are cold, we should drink less green tea and reduce our fruit intake to every other day, until we start to warm up again. You will notice that this naturally starts to happen in wintertime, when most people find themselves less inclined to want to eat fruit. In summertime the opposite happens, the body and mind seems to be encouraging us to have more and more of it to help us cool down.

We cannot assume anything about a fruit or any other food until we have tasted it. When a fruit is not ripe it will be very bitter. The more it ripens in the sun the sweeter it will usually get. For example, grapes will start with very bitter properties, but as they ripen they will develop sweetness with an undercurrent or aftertaste of bitterness. This is recognisable as although you may have tasted sweet initially, your mouth has been left dry after eating them. When you get more than one flavour in a food, you must figure out the likely outcome of the combination. Here sweetness builds energy and helps power up the detoxifying effect in a gentle way. However, if the grapes were left to over ripen they would eventually lose the bitter effect altogether. So we must always judge the effects of the food on its intensity of flavour and not just on the family it belongs to.

Plants and trees produce these flavours in nature for very clever reasons. Firstly they don't want their fruits to be eaten until they have matured the seeds inside of them. So to start with they are very bitter and off putting. They act like natural pesticides. When the seeds are ready they use the suns' natural energies to ripen and sweeten the fruit. However, they often retain a bitter undercurrent and the seeds too can be more bitter. If you have ever eaten grapes with seeds, you will notice the harsh bitterness when you bite down on them. After birds and animals have eaten this now ripe fruit, the remaining bitterness causes fluid to gather in the intestines and helps to wash the seeds quickly down through the intestines and out of the animals. The seeds are then deposited in a new area, where fresh life can burst forth and begin its journey.

When herbs are harvested in China, it is essential to taste and then pick them at certain times to ensure they have the right properties to be used in medicines. If they are gathered at the wrong time, they will not have the right action and must be discarded.

Bitter foods can often be helpful to the heart and cardiovascular system. As they are good at purging fats and toxins from the body and in this case the blood vessels. They can help to lower your cholesterol, just like the way statins are used in Western Medicine. By clearing any blockages from the blood vessels, you are less likely to suffer a heart attack or stroke. Also, because the heart does not have to push as hard to get the blood through all those narrowed vessels filled with cholesterol, it can preserve its power, strength and energy. And will in effect, last longer.

The Sour Flavour.

The main characteristics of sour is that it astringes, tightens, locks and holds in. It initially has the same reaction as bitterness. The cells tighten away from it and squeeze fluid out. However sourness continues to hold this tightness for some time. In your mouth, after tasting bitter, it will tighten, water, relax and go dry. With sourness it will be held in that tight state and stay moist.

This has several implications in the body. It can tighten and tone up muscles and hold them and organs in place. It can stop fluids leaking from the body, such as sweat leaking from the pores. This can also lock down the body, making it harder for bacteria to enter. It can help with dry coughs and asthma, by holding fluids into the lungs and lubricating them. It can moisten and preserve nutrients and cells in the body, just like pickles preserved in a jar of sour vinegar. It can help to hold hormones and fluids in blood, making it stronger.

In mild amounts it can help to gently cleanse and detoxify organs like the liver. However, in big amounts sourness tends to over tighten and strangle processes in the body, causing muscular problems and organs to seize up and stop working properly. Even our minds can feel uptight and become stressed. For this reason, it is important not to over indulge in sour foods if you are stressed and under pressure. When overused it tends to choke up our livers and prevent them from functioning. So we must always be careful to use the sour flavour in small doses.

The Spicy Flavour.

Also commonly referred to as pungent or aromatic. It is characterized by having and creating a feeling of movement through the mouth and body. If you smell these foods, their strong aromas will feel as if they are shooting up through your head. In the mouth they often cause a tingling, racing, rushing sensation. In the body they do several things. Firstly, as they intermingle with other parts of you and excite and agitate your cells, they can cause movement and activity. This generates energy and heat, just the same as if you were to start exercising and moving a lot you would end up getting hot. Spices therefore generally warm you up. There are exceptions, one such is peppermint, which has a mix of moving and cooling properties to produce both a fiery and a cool draughty sensation.

Because of all this moving, heating, drying and pushing, spices are very useful at dealing with dampness and phlegm. They can be used to clear phlegm from the digestion, lungs, nose, sinus and head in particular. By drying fluids from the digestion it can prevent them from being absorbed and causing fluid retention in other parts of the body.

Be warned however, if you have phlegm, sometimes spices can initially seem like they are worsening your symptoms. As phlegm is pushed and forced up on top of itself, it can make you feel as if you are more blocked up. So you should start with mild amounts of spicy herbs to stop big build ups. And then give it time to slowly work the phlegm out of you. Obviously, you will want to cut back on damp and phlegm forming foods as well.

By moving blood and energy, spices help circulation around the body. This is nearly like exercising internally. They can speed up your metabolism. Make foods move more quickly through your intestines. Burn up nutrients, food and fats, dry fluids and help you lose weight. They can have a very strong effect on the lungs by not only clearing fluids from them but by also giving them energy to breathe more effectively. They can cause your pores to open which can be useful to allow excess from the body, to help push out bacteria and viruses. And is even used by some, particularly in India, to open pores and let heat out in summertime to cool the body down. I personally prefer other methods, which we will discuss shortly, for keeping the body cool.

In excess spices can cause some major problems. All that heat can burn up your energy, leaving you feeling tired and eventually exhausting you. It can also burn up your blood and nutrients, dry out your skin and hair, and damage all parts of you. If your pores are left open, you can lose energy, and fluids from your blood and vital essences as well. The heat from the spices can also expand your blood which can lead to ruptures, easy bleeding, skin rashes, high blood pressure and even strokes. The most serious common problem, however, is when heat combines with phlegm and toxins. This deadly mix can lead to many uncomfortable ailments and potentially very serious illnesses. More will be explained when we discuss heating foods.

The Salty Taste.

Its characteristics are to cool, as it is a mineral, which will be explained shortly. And to move, clean, moisten, soften, astringe and preserve. When we put it in our mouths we notice a couple of things. Firstly it gently tingles and fizzes. It's causing molecules to move. It also attracts and astringes moisture. So you are left with a wet mouth after tasting it. If we were to leave a small pile of salt on a plate in a cold and damp room, when we come back to it the next day, we will find a little pool of salty water. The salt will have drawn moisture from the air into itself. In the body, salt will hold onto fluids passing through it and keep the cells it is interacting with moist.

Our tears are salty and our sweat is salty too. This stops these areas from drying out. If you did not have salt, your eyes would not be able to remain lubricated. Salt is found in many places throughout the body. The brain is kept in a salty liquid. As babies we are formed in a bag of salty fluid.

As it has the ability to astringe, it can be used to fortify and lock and hold fluids into the body. It can help build the blood and also retain hormones, in particular those related to the kidneys, reproductive and adrenal glands. In this way, by preserving these precious essences, it can help to slow down aging. By moistening and cooling the skin and other areas, it can stop them from drying out and reduce wrinkles. However, beware, if you put salt onto your skin, it will draw fluids from it. Salt must be digested and caught up inside your body to start to retain fluids that can help you. And if you do not take in sufficient fluids, salt can hold onto what you do have and start to dry you out internally, so be sure to consume some fluids with the salt in your diet.

A type of salty seaweed is sometimes used in Chinese herbal medicine to soften lumps and tumours. As salt pulls moisture into it, when it mingles with cells, it pulls moisture to itself and ends up also moistening these cells around it. Salt also fizzes and causes movement.

You can imagine the effect if you leave salty water on a dried out grimy pot. After a while, the grime will soften as it absorbs the moisture. And the molecules in the grime aided by the movement of the salt will start to break up and disperse. You will then find it very easy to wash the pot clean. Bleach is a component of salt. And other chemicals from salt are often used in common soaps and detergents. So salty foods and herbs can be used to break and soften unwanted masses in the body.

We can even see salt corroding and rusting the bottoms of cars when it has been used to de-ice roads after snowfalls. Salt does not heat snow up, but it does start to move its' molecules. Turning it from ice into water. Salty water has a much lower freezing point than water. In the body, salt because of the movement can stimulate energy but as it also has a heavy mineral, it will cool and not cause you to heat up. Obviously because it cools and retains fluids, salt is better for you in hot dry climates and not so good in cold wet winters.

Overuse of salt can overcool the body and cause it to retain too much fluid. Particularly affecting the lower body, the kidneys, hips, knees, legs, ankles and feet. It can also in overuse, pull too much fluid into our bloodstream, causing it to expand and increase pressure on our blood vessels. This in turn over time affects and weakens our hearts and kidneys by causing too much pressure and stress on them.

In general if you have a good natural diet, you need to add salt into it as required. But if you eat lots of processed food, you will probably find, you are actually over consuming salt, as many of these products have too much added during their manufacture.

The Sweet Taste.

The main characteristic is its stickiness. In nature it is usually formed from the suns effect on plants. The more energy and heat that fruits and sugar cane get from the sun, the more ripe and more sweet tasting they end up being. Because of this, when it is consumed sugar itself can release into the body the stored energy it has taken from the sun.

However there is a second and equally important way that sugar causes energy in our bodies. And that is through friction. Anything that blocks the movement of particles through your body or impedes the actions of organs causes them to power up and try to force their activity through. As they release and use more energy to push through the stickiness, our bodies start to heat up and rev up our existing energy systems.

When we eat sweet foods, we get a sugar rush. And while this high lasts, we will feel pretty good. However, the problem is, that it is now using up our existing energy supplies and leaving a sticky, gooey, nasty mess inside of us. So, if we take too much sweet stuff in, we can expect to receive a sugar high followed by a slump and a low. Also the sticky mess left behind can cause phlegm and toxins to get trapped and rot and decay amongst our cells, tissues and organs. This can obviously lead to many unpleasant and dangerous ills.

Sugar in moderation, that is small amounts of naturally sweet foods, not over processed sugars, can be helpful to the body. It can gently strengthen our energy. In particular boosting our digestive powers to break down foods. Because it is sticky it can also slow down the movement of good healthy foods through our digestive tract, allowing it to have more time to break down these foods and pull all the good nutrients and further energy from them, to fortify our bodies.

Summary Of The Five Flavours.

The bitter taste detoxifies. It cools, cleans and purges. In large or unbalanced doses it can wash too much from your system, leaving you weak and drained.

The bitter taste causes your mouth to clench and tighten up. Then to moisten and flush the bitterness away and finally to relax and feel dry.

Examples of bitter foods are pineapple, rhubarb, pomegranate, cranberry, unripe grapes and green tea.

The sour taste astringes. It holds, moistens and locks in nutrients. It seals the body from outer threats. In small amounts it can help to break up fats and cleanse. If you take too much it can strangle your system, block it up and even make you feel more stressed.

The sour taste causes your mouth to clench just like the bitter taste. But then it holds it tight for much longer. It tends to leave your mouth wet and seized up.

Examples of sour foods are vinegar, onions, cider and some types of apples and their juices.

The spicy taste moves, heats, expectorates and dries. It can enhance circulation and speed up metabolism, driving fluids and phlegm out through your lungs and pores. If you take too much you can start to over heat. This heat can congeal and thicken phlegm and toxins, which can lead to very dangerous illnesses. The heat can also burn out your energy and exhaust you.

The spicy taste causes lots of movement and activity in your mouth. And will either make it hot like when you eat chilli or cold and hot like when you eat peppermint.

Examples of spicy foods are garlic, chilli, turmeric, ginger, mustard, curry, and green or red peppers.

The sweet taste in small amounts can build our energy. If over used it can create toxins and leave a nasty sticky sludge in our bodies, which will block them up. This can cause heat to build up and can wear out our good energy and make us tired.

The sweet taste leaves your mouth feeling sticky and gooey.

Examples of sweet foods are honey, raw cane sugar, dates, sun dried raisins, peas and ripe bananas.

The salty taste astringes fluids. It gently cools, moves, cleans, moistens, softens and preserves. In large amounts, it can swell our blood and create too much pressure in it and our organs. It can cause fluid retention in the body.

The salty taste leaves your mouth feeling wet and tingling.

Examples of salty foods are salt, oysters and sea food, seaweed and fish.

Neutral tastes tend to have the action of fortifying the body. They tend to be more like the building blocks inside of us. They can become part of the body and be accepted without any agitation to it. Foods like rice can build and strengthen both energy and blood. A neutral food as its taste increases will start to fall into one of the five flavours, so traditionally, it is not seen as separate from them. Rice would be seen as a very weak version of the Sweet Flavour.

Do also note that a food can have more than one flavour which can cause it to have more than one action. A simple example would be an apple. This can be both sweet and sour. The sweetness will create energy and the sourness will lock and hold in fluids. Apples also contain minerals which will provide a cooling quality to their nature.

You can start to see how we can use all these flavours to balance our bodies and to change their overall patterns. It is important to remember that the stronger the flavour or aroma, the stronger the reaction will be in the body. Think of comparing a cup of mildly bitter green tea with a cup of intensely bitter lemon juice. The lemon juice, if you can manage to drink a whole cup of it, will have your mouth and face all screwed up and you may even get a stomach ache as it clamps up your insides.

By the extreme reactions that some foods can cause, you can see the power that they have to treat and change conditions in the body. Another example is a chilli pepper. Try eating a small handful to see how hot you get. A cold person by having a little amount on a daily basis will start to heat parts of themselves up and alter their internal states. This leads us to the next chapter in which we will discuss hot and cold foods.

Chapter Nineteen - Hot And Cold Foods.

First off, we are not talking about the physical temperature of these foods and fluids. What we are talking about is the reactions they cause in the human body that generate some form of internal heat or cold.

Heat Inducing Foods.

It is very easy to see heat produced from foods we eat, because we quite quickly heat up after eating them. Heat acts rapidly in nature, whereas cold tends to follow a more slow trend. If we were to put our hands near fire, we feel it instantly and pull our hands away. But with cold, we could quite easily keep our hand in a freezer for ten or more minutes before it becomes painfully cold. In the body we get the same picture from hot and cold foods. Heating foods tend to heat us immediately. Whereas cooling foods, slowly cool us down over a period of hours, days or even months.

The most common heating foods are coffee, red or black tea, spices, alcohol, fats and sugars. If you took chilled whiskey from the fridge, poured it into a cold glass filled with ice cubes and then knocked it back, you would still very quickly feel the burning in your throat and the heat spreading across your chest. It's easy to see this heating effect. These foods warm your body and release and excite the energy within it. They can give you power to strengthen organs, mind and spirit. They speed things up and generally stimulate the body. They are good for improving mood and vitality.

The down side is, they use your nutrients up to do this. Just as petrol poured onto a fire increase flames, and quickly burns up the logs. Hot food increases your energy, and then burns up your stores and reserves of nutrients. Eventually if you really over indulge, it will even start to burn up your tissues and hormones, emaciating you and making you age more quickly.

The best way to use these hot activating stimulants is to combine them with food. For example, if you drink alcohol by itself it will burn up your nutrients and reserves. Giving you a temporary high but leaving you to crash afterwards. If however you have a small amount of alcohol with a meal, then it will boost your digestion helping you to fully break down and retrieve all the nutrients from the food. It may burn up some of these in the process but you should be left overall with a net gain in terms of both fresh energy and reserves.

Another nasty thing they can do is heat and cook phlegm, fluids and toxins causing serious disorders. You can easily see this through an example of a fry up on a pan. If you have it on a mild setting, the food cooks slowly but evenly. You may get fats and oils oozing from the sausages and bacon, but they will stay in a more soft and liquid form on the mild heat. However, if you turn the heat up too high, everything starts to burn, the fats in particular will congeal and turn into a hardened black tar. I am sure you are aware, it's easy to wash the soft fats and greases off the pan with your bitter flavoured washing up liquid. But if it has turned into these sticky hard blackened lumps, it will take hours and hours of emersion in water and soap to soften and remove them. If you overheat your body, all phlegm, fluids and fats start to congeal, thicken and rot. Embedding themselves amongst your healthy cells and continuing to decompose, they will cause harm and destruction all around.

As we discussed in the five flavours chapter, there are a few ways to generate heat in the body from food. Spices, pungent and aromatic flavours move energy, causing molecules to vibrate more and generate heat inside of you. And sugars release stored energy from the sun which gives heat but also their stickiness binds to things trying to move through your body and function in it. This causes them to rev up and push harder thus generating even more heat.

Cold Inducing Foods.

We must remember that cold acts much more slowly and far less obviously than heat. If you consume a cooling food now, it will take a few hours before you would notice any effect. Because of this, the mind does not usually associate the food as being responsible for cooling the system. But when you become conscious of this and know how to look for it, you will see that these cooling foods really are having this effect.

There are two methods we can use to cool the body through foods. We have already encountered one, the bitter flavour. This is particularly useful when phlegm and toxins are present. Bitterness expels and purges, and as it pushes away obstructions from the circulation and your organs, you will find that everything is moving more freely and therefore needs less energy to keep it moving. As energy slows the heat it produces diminishes and the body cools. In excess, bitter can even start to push the nutrients out that feed the energy. This causes a further cooling. In summertime, we are naturally drawn to more bitter fruit to cool ourselves down.

The second and main way we cool down our bodies is through heavy dense cooling particles in our foods. Like heavy proteins and minerals. About five percent of our body is composed of minerals. They help in lots of functions in the body. One of them is in cooling. In nature, a general rule, is that the more dense something gets the more cold it feels. When you put your hand on feathers, then wood, then cement, then steel, you will notice the harder, heavier, more dense they are, the cooler they appear to be. Your dense heavy mineral filled bones will be much cooler than the surrounding flesh and blood. In physics, they would tell you that what is really happening, is if something appears to be cold, it is pulling energy from you. When it appears to be hot, it is emitting energy to you. We can see the effective use of this principle all around us. In our clothes, ultra light and thin materials are used for ski wear. Carpets are used in cold climates to warm floors, and tiles in hot ones to keep them cool. Even houses made of stone are used in hot countries compared to houses made of wood in the colder ones.

When we consume heavy foods, laden with minerals, they are broken down and pulled into our bodies. Vegetables are an excellent source, probably the best. But cooling particles can be found in most types of food, even in water. When you look at a bottle of water it seems crystal clear, but in fact, as you read the label on the back of the bottle, you will find that it is filled with many minerals. The particles are so small they are not visible to the naked eye. You will notice that if you touch a bottle of water, it always seems cooler than the temperature of the room it is in. Water beds get so cold that even in hot places like California, people cannot sleep on them unless they are heated up. If you are over heating in a hot summer you can fill up a couple of old plastic bottles with water and put them in your bed. You will find at night, that they will cool it and you down.

When we eat vegetables, water or anything else containing minerals and proteins, these tiny particles get deposited throughout our bodies. They mix amongst our cells. And as living things move and create energy, some of their heat is pulled away into these cooler minerals. This stops the cells from over heating and suffering any damage.

The dense heavy particles don't use up the energy they are pulling away from the living bodily cells, they merely store it. Once the active cells start to lose power and their temperature drops below the energy stored in the mineral, then the mineral will start to feed this energy stored in them back to the cells until there is balance once again.

You can see this working very simply outside the body. If you put your warm hand on a cold radiator or other metal object. Energy will start to be transferred from you into it. After a few minutes, if you take your hand away, then get someone to touch that area. They will notice it is warm compared to everywhere else on the radiator. Literally the cold metal has soaked up and drained energy from you into it. It will now feed that energy back into the room until it becomes cool again.

When you consistently eat your vegetables and gather these cooling elements into the body, you will eventually notice your whole system seems to be cooling down. This is usually good and will slow down ageing and preserve your body and cells. Just like the way a fridge slows down the deterioration of your food and instead keeps it nice and fresh. There have been multiple studies linking vegetables to the slowing down of aging and the extending of life.

However, be aware that you can have too much vegetables and overcool your body, leading to a lack of energy and power. This may over time produce cold type illnesses. In the past, in Western society, most people remember seeing some vegetarians who looked tired, drained and lifeless.

Often with dull, pasty complexions. They had simply consumed too many vegetables, which created too much cold in their bodies and slowed all their functioning down. There are many vegetarians in India, China and throughout Asia who get around this overcooling by adding hot spices into food to create more balanced meals.

Summary Of Hot And Cold Inducing Foods.

In summary, foods like alcohol, coffee, spices, red and black teas, that cause activity and movement also generate heat. Foods that are sticky like sugar and fats release stored energy into the body to warm it, but more often impede the circulation and activity of organs. Causing them to rev up and push harder, thus generating heat as a by product.

Foods that are bitter, cool by counteracting stickiness and allowing freer movement. As organs have to work less they cool down. Bitter flavours can also flush nutrients that fuel energy which causes less of it and heat to be created in the first place. The long term method of cooling the body is to eat and retain cooling particles found in minerals and heavy proteins in foods like vegetables, beans and nuts.

Chapter Twenty - Dryness, Dampness, Phlegm And Toxins.

In this chapter we will discuss a few more categories our foods can fit into. We will start with dryness.

Dryness.

It usually comes from three areas. Firstly we have the bitter taste, which pushes fluids out from the body. Over consumption of these can start to deplete your internal fluids. Excessive consumption of intense bitter tastes like lemon, lime and grapefruit can quickly drain fluids over a week or two. For example, they can start to dry your skin, and weaken your blood. With less blood, oxygen and nutrients to the brain your mood will also start to lower.

Heat is the next variable that dries. Like a hot sun in summertime, it quickly burns, evaporates and uses up fluids. Leaving you thirsty and dehydrated.

And finally dryness can come from not eating enough cooling minerals and heavy dense nutrients. If you are not taking in enough of these and cooling moistening substances. Your body will eventually go out of balance and become too hot and dry.

Dampness And Phlegm.

Dampness refers to watery fluids and phlegm refers to heavier more congealed sticky fluids. In the body they can get in the way of circulation and processes, blocking things up and slowing them down.

Fresh fluids in the body usually start out clear or white, they may be cool or hot in nature. If they are heated and cooked over time they turn yellowy and darker. If they are cooled they tend to stay clear or white and become thick and heavy.

The foods that produce cold, damp and phlegm in our bodies tend to be sweet tasting and heavy mineral based ones. The heavy mineral ones, as described earlier, tend to create cold and reduce energy. Which in turn, congeals and thickens fluids, just as we see the cold creating fluids in winter, where everything gets wet and damp.

Too much sweet fruit can also create damp in the body. Whereas bitter fruit pushes fluid away, sweet sticky fruit can actually help cold fluids gather. We see this in bananas and mangoes and so forth. They are cooling and heavy in minerals by nature, but are also mildly sweet. So when you bite on one, you find your mouth gets very moist and gooey on the inside. Imagine comparing a bitter lemon, which leaves your mouth dry, to a banana which leaves it feeling like you have a slimy goo on the inside of it.

Another common creator of damp and phlegm is a cold and weak digestive system. If your body has weak energy. It will not have sufficient power to fully break down food and drink. This may lead to large amounts of fluids and phlegm being created when you eat.

Foods that are rich and hard to digest can also cause damp and phlegm. The most well known of these foods is dairy (which will be discussed in detail later). If you overeat, then most types of food can actually lead to undigested particles forming damp and phlegm inside of you. These will clog you. They may become cold or hot dependant on the other conditions in the rest of your body.

There is also one other method to create damp and phlegm in the body. This is through the ingestion of physically cold drinks and meals (This will also be discussed in detail later).

Damp and phlegm commonly tire our bodies, as they waste precious energy trying to clean and dry up the excess moisture.

Damp Heat, Hot Phlegm And Toxins.

Damp heat and hot phlegm can be created by mixing rich energetic foods and heating foods. For example, oils, grease, animal fats and sugary sticky foods. These foods by themselves can generate damp and heat because they are sticky and gooey and can bind to and over activate your energy which heats and ferments them, turning them into a nasty slime. Imagine yellow and green phlegm or odorous runny sticky bowel movement.

When you start bringing heating foods like alcohol, spices and coffee into this mix it becomes even more hot and foul. If heat becomes really excessive it will burn these fluids into a nasty tar like substance. Think of burning fats until they are like a black glue on to a frying pan. At this stage the phlegm has now become toxic.

We can also get toxins through our diets from burnt foods. Burnt food may be tasty but cannot be digested. It only creates problems, difficulties and harm in the body. Many Western studies have linked burnt and barbecued foods to cancer. It should be avoided wherever possible. Toxins can also come from the many preservatives, additives and chemicals now dumped into our foods and even through the over processing of the food itself.

Another pattern that often causes toxins is an overheated digestive system. If someone suffers from an overheated stomach, which can give symptoms like heartburn, repeating, and feelings of food being stuck in that area. Then the intense stomach heat can burn food in it and hold it there for too long, overcooking it and turning it to phlegm. The intestines too can become dirty and over heated. As good clean food enters, it mixes with this turbid mess and the whole lot is contaminated.

Obviously, the presence of damp heat, hot phlegm and toxins in our bodies is a most unwelcome one. It is the cause of most modern Western illnesses. It often shows its presence through unpleasant odours and dark yellow fluids emitted from the body. If you have these signs you need to reduce phlegm creating substances and add in natural detoxifiers but beware, toxins can take years to build up in your system. Many people have been gathering them since childhood. If this is the case, don't expect them to go away in a week, a month or even a year. I have seen it take as much as five years for some people to clean their systems after many years, even decades of eating a toxic diet.

Summary Of Dry, Damp, Phlegm And Toxic Creating Foods.

Dryness can come from the bitter taste pushing too much fluid from your body. From heat drying fluids up. Or from a lack of cooling minerals which keep things moist.

Dampness and phlegm usually come from too much cold in our systems. The cold will usually come from ingesting too many cooling foods or from physically cold food and drink. It may also come from something that has weakened our energy and generally cooled us down.

Pre-existing heat in our bodies or the over consumption of foods that our hot in nature like coffee and alcohol, when mixed with thick fluids, phlegm producing foods like dairy or man made chemicals can also lead to the production of damaging hot phlegm and toxins.

Chapter Twenty One   -   Putting It All Together.

So far we have learnt about the five flavours - bitter, sour, spicy, salty and sweet. We have discussed the active nature of foods - hot and cold, drying and moistening. How can all this help us ? The answer is once again through balancing our bodies. To keep it simple …

If we are too cold, we eat foods that heat us up.
If we are too hot, we eat foods that cool us down.
If we are too dry, we eat foods that moisten us and create fluid.
If we are too damp, we eat foods that disperse and dry the damp away.

In this way we can balance ourselves, change the internal patterns in our bodies, heal many illnesses and create good health.

On top of the internal conditions that we have, we must also continuously adapt and change to external events in our lives. When the weather changes, we don't need to just change our clothes but our foods as well. If we overwork or exercise we need more and different foods. If we get stressed or any other emotional state, we again can change this through our foods.

There is no food or drink from nature that is good or bad for you. It is all dependant on what is already going on in your body. For example, if you are cold, then alcohol, coffee and spices can warm you up and bring you back into a balanced healthy state, not too hot and not too cold. Where everything works well. However if its ninety degrees outside and your sweltering in the heat. Then even a little coffee and alcohol can cause you to burn up, which may create considerable damage internally. When I eat now, I always go for balance. If I am cold, I will go to the press and add spices to my meal to cause extra heat. If I am too hot I will go too the fridge and drink fruit juice to cool myself down.

What your body needs today, it may not need tomorrow. You must constantly factor this in and change it as is appropriate. When you think of Western dietary guides, you see how rigid and fixed they are. X grams of this vitamin, Y grams of that mineral. X amount of calories daily for men and Y amount for women and so on. You can easily see that this is wrong because we are all different shapes, and sizes. That it is also wrong because we live in different climates, do different amounts and types of work, have different emotional backgrounds, different lifestyles and of course are different ages. Everything constantly moves and changes. And our diets must move and change with us too.

In Practical Useful Terms We Can Balance Things Using These Methods ...

Too much heat and dryness - Reduce heating and drying foods like spices, alcohol, coffee, red and black teas. Eat more cooling and moistening foods and fluids filled with heavy minerals and substances. Such as most vegetables, (excluding spicy peppers and onions). In particular sea vegetables and also sweet and sour moistening fruit like orange juice, mango, pear, apple and banana. Also make sure you have adequate salt in your diet.

Too much heat and phlegm - Reduce heating and drying foods like spices, alcohol, coffee, dark chocolate, red and black teas. Reduce phlegm and toxic foods like sweets, cakes, sugars, dairy, greases, milk chocolate, fats, overly processed and burnt foods. Then eat cooling and clearing foods. Such as pomegranates, grapes and berries. Drink lots of green tea. If you have infections, drink lemon, lime or grapefruit in water once a day for a couple of weeks. Then take a break from it for a few days, and repeat if necessary. Also add salt if there is not enough in your diet.

Too much cold and dryness - Temporarily reduce your intake of fruit and vegetables. Add small quantities of sour foods to retain fluids, like vinegar and apple. Increase intake of fluids in the form of hot sweet drinks. And add small amounts of spice to warm you up.

Too much cold and damp or phlegm - Temporarily reduce your intake of fruit and vegetables. Add heating and drying foods such as coffee, alcohol and spices to your meals. Add small amounts of sweet food as well. And add drying foods such as white rice.

If undernourished and weak - Add more sweet foods to gently build you up. White rice is considered a balanced mildly sweet food in Chinese Medicine. It is excellent for building energy and blood and strengthening digestion. Also add sour foods to lock in the nutrients you are digesting. Also add nuts, seeds and eggs to your diet. They will boost your hormones and will generally fortify the body.

If stressed - Add more cooling foods to reduce the heat that the impact of the stress on your body is producing. Avoid all sour foods, like apples, vinegar and onions. These will tighten your body in a similar way to how stress tightens it. Add peppermint as it gently moves blocked energy and relaxes the flow of nutrients through your muscles. Good oils will also reverse the damage the tightening effect of stress does. They will help everything move more freely and smoothly through your system. And add sweet food to build the body and blood and nutrients to the brain, to help it think clearly and calmly.

Below Are A Few Little Points To Note When You Are Trying To Balance The Body.

Firstly, remember that as flavours become stronger, they will increase in potency and have more dramatic effects on your system. It is always best to start small and slowly increase intensity until the required level is met. If you try to push things too fast you can cause a new imbalance. In particular if you add strong stimulants like coffee, red and black tea, alcohol and spices in large amounts, you can quickly imbalance the body. If you think of petrol on a fire, you can see a little of a stimulant can have a very big effect.

If you are trying to cool your body. Be careful that you don't overcool and over power your digestive organs before the rest of the body is done. The digestion needs a certain amount of energy and therefore heat to break down your food and extract nutrients from it. The more heavy and cold the nutrients, the more energy it needs to do the job. So if you are eating something with lots of cooling minerals, like vegetables, make sure you eat something that creates energy and power with it, like rice and a small amount of mild spices like garlic or mustard seed.

When preparing a meal, it is a good idea to start with a bland food like rice. Then add small amounts of other flavours. Avoid any really intense flavours unless you are purposely trying to alter an out of sync state in your body. For example, hot spicy curries are not a good idea unless you are freezing cold. Rather than making spicy dishes, you are better to add small pinches when cooking meals to season them. And then after they are done, you can add extra at the dining table if you think they need a little more as you are eating them.

When your body is healthy and balanced. It is best to take small amounts of each flavour everyday. This keeps all the organs stimulated and in good working order.

Also be sure to take in a large variety of different foods. Foods can be light, heavy or in-between. They can have fine easily broken down particles or thick heavy ones. Because of this they will break down into different areas in the body. And primarily cause their effects in those areas. In order for all parts of the body to be healthy we need a wide selection of foods. For example, with the bitter taste, bitter cranberries are very good for cleaning and cooling the kidneys and the bladder, whereas bitter grapes more so clean the intestines.

Examples Of Some Good And Bad Food Combinations.

Coffee and cake would be very bad, as the heat will burn and tar up the fats and sugars in the cake, creating toxins. If you must eat cake or sweets, you would be better to combine it with bitter fruit or juice like pomegranate or even lemon, as they will break up the fats in the cake. And also the bitterness will cause your cells to tighten, release fluids and push away the fats and sugars from the cake.

Coffee and milk creates heat, phlegm and toxins. Whereas weak black coffee which heats and dries followed by an orange juice which cools and moistens, would nearly balance each other.

Salad and water creates too much cold and may overwhelm digestive organs, reducing their energy and power. If constantly repeated you may end up slowing and weakening your metabolism, which may cause you to retain fluids and gain weight. Add a hot drink or rice or peppers and spice to the salad to balance it.

Finally, remember that it is not just about putting good foods into your diet but also about taking the bad stuff out. Start with small changes and over time, even if it takes years, you will manage to modify your diet without any real hardship. You will see the gains as you do this, but also remember what you are not seeing as well. What you won't see or feel, is the pain and the suffering from all the illnesses you would have most likely encountered if you had stayed on an unhealthy diet.

Chapter Twenty Two - The Workings Of The Digestive System.

Firstly we have the mouth. The mouth chomps, cuts and breaks down our food into smaller more digestible pieces. It combines it with saliva which starts the digestive process. It is very important to really chew your food. The more you chew, the less energy your stomach will have to waste trying to break down the food. Teeth can do the work so much easier than your stomach can. Make sure you particularly chew meats, beans, nuts and tough types of food. Using chopsticks is a good idea, as it slows down the amount of food getting into and the rate at which it gets delivered to your mouth. Allowing you to chew and even savour and enjoy the taste of your food more.

Next Up Is The Stomach.

When food enters the stomach, the digestive system heats up and releases digestive enzymes to break it down. This is comparable to cooking food on a stove. Digestive energy and enzymes can reach burning temperatures. The stomach itself has a mucus protective lining which stops its own cells from being burnt up. If you have ever experienced heartburn, you have gotten a taste of how hot it gets in your stomach.

One of the golden rules of Chinese Dietary Therapy is to always heat your food and drink. Always avoid physically cold food and drinks. The nature of the stomach is to heat up to break down food. Therefore anytime you put anything cold into it, you are going against its nature and draining away its vital energy and power to perform. Eating cold food and drink is the most inefficient way of digesting your food.

If you could imagine cooking frozen vegetables in icy cold water. And then for some mad reason, just as it starts to boil to add ice cubes in, you can see that this way the cooker will use and waste lots of electricity. Now compare this to boiling the kettle, getting it to use the energy instead, adding thawed unfrozen vegetables to the pot and then putting the boiled water in on top. This way the cooker has used the least amount of electricity.

This is the same inside our bodies. If we put cold food into our stomach and wash it down with icy drinks, it is squandering and wasting our precious energy. The stomach and intestines will then often have to steal energy from the rest of our body to complete the job of digestion, making us feel tired and sleepy after a meal. On top of that, food will not be broken down properly. So we don't get the full compliment of energy and nutrients from it. This also leaves heavier undigested particles in our system, which often create damp, phlegm or sludge. To correct this, all we need to do is to heat our meals and have physically hot drinks with them.

Even fruit juice in winter should be consumed at room temperature or warm and not freezing cold from the fridge. This is easily accomplished by adding some hot water from the kettle to it. You can even add more if you wish, to turn your fruit juices into a tea.

Cooking foods as opposed to eating them raw is also better for you, as the heat helps to start softening and breaking down your food. But don't overcook or burn your food, as this can waste and damage the nutrients.

We can also add mild stimulants to our meals to help digest them, as they encourage movement, heat and activity. These include small amounts of spices, alcohol, weak coffee, red or black tea. But be sure not to add too many, as you can turn the heat in your stomach into a raging fire causing heartburn and other ills.

Stomach Problems.

When the stomach overheats from too much heating foods like alcohol, coffee and spices. Or from eating sticky, rich, greasy foods which block it up and cause too much heat to build up, such as sugars, cakes, fry ups, sweets and dairy. You may start to get symptoms like heartburn, bad breath, toothache, bleeding gums, mouth ulcers, gum disease, hiccups, repeating, belching, ulcers, vomiting, regurgitation and feelings of fullness or pain in the stomach area. The heat may even agitate the mind, making it race and causing anxiety, irritability and sleeping problems.

Poor sleep can also often be caused by eating late at night. This causes your stomach to overheat the blood, heart and head creating too much activity and restless sleep.

Eating late at night can also develop a pattern of general overheating of the stomach as well. The stomach like the rest of us needs time to rest and cool down. So keeping it going at night steals this precious recuperative time.

Obviously you should avoid eating at night. However some bitter fruit or juices, or green or peppermint teas can be helpful when consumed in the evening. Because they are bitter, the stomach pushes them very quickly through it, washing it as they go. Leaving it clean, ready and fresh for the next day. They can also cool and settle you down, preparing you for sleep.

To keep a clean and well running digestive tract, you should always have green and peppermint teas (its properties will be discussed later), after meals and between them. Then add in bitter fruit juices for extra cleaning and cooling, as and when you think you need them. This is similar to washing your pans, pots and plates after meals. You certainly would not try to re-use dirty pots and dishes again. Equally so, try to clean up the digestive tract after each meal.

Heat and phlegm generally cause stomach problems like heartburn and queasiness but two other factors can also come into play. Harsh cold can cramp and seize the stomach and when combined with bitterness can cause heartburn. The stomach spasms tightly on the inside, pops the flap from the food pipe open and heat and enzymes escape up it burning your throat. This will never happen if you avoid eating cold food and drinks.

The other factor is a much more common one and that is stress. Stress again causes tightness. This can buckle the stomach and intestines, causing foods to get trapped in them. Which can lead to heat and gasses building up as the food continues to rot and ferment, giving heartburn, bloating and sometimes painful indigestion.

This trapped food when it overheats in the intestines, may lead to damp heat and phlegm forming in them. This can produce gas and odorous foul smelling rotten stools. The vicious circle of stress will also allow poisons and toxins to enter and build up in your body and impede the release and breakdown of good nutrients, leaving your organs and brain deficient in them. Often causing the mind to worry more and preventing it from achieving the calmness and clarity, needed to deal with the stress in the first place.

The Intestines.

This is a really long tube ending in your colon. In an adult it can be from twenty to over thirty feet long. It further breaks down the food and absorbs it into the bloodstream through villi, which are like tiny little fingers sucking nutrients in and then moving the rest of the food along. It then sends the waste and leftovers down through the colon and out of the body.

Again we can see that heat and cold create the big patterns affecting the workings of the intestines. Starting with cold, it quite simply slows everything down. As power is diminished, food is left undigested leading to a build up of phlegm and fluids in the intestines and throughout the rest of the body. As they are beside each other cold can travel to and particularly affect the kidneys. It also badly affects the lungs, by dumping large amounts of damp and phlegm created from improperly digested foods into them for exhalation.

In the intestines themselves, as there is no energy to break down and move foods, you will find they gather and start to block you up. This can cause distension, bloating, indigestion, gurgling, gas, cramps, sluggish and loose bowel movements with little or no odour.

You may also get dull achy lower back pain, copious amounts of clear urine and swollen ankles if the kidneys have insufficient power and energy to efficiently filter blood and fluids.

You may have lots of clear or white phlegm in the lungs or in the sinus and nose. Most nasal congestion can be resolved through the avoidance of cold diets and phlegm producing diets. Unfortunately for me, I spent most of my childhood suffering from a blocked stuffy nose. After repeated visits to the doctor, I was put on a steroid nasal spray. I had to use it twice every day. And even with that, it still only produced limited effects, clearing about half the mucus away. When I began learning Chinese Medicine, I gave up dairy products and my nose cleared by 90 percent. I happily threw the steroid spray away. And after the introduction of heating foods to my diet, my digestive system stopped producing phlegm and now my nose remains fully clear.

Other effects from a cold digestive system can be seen in the head and body. As phlegm gathers in your brain, it blocks up all the little connections. This can lead to poor memory and concentration. To people appearing to be blank, lost for words and even dopey. The mind when not receiving enough nutrients from the proper breakdown of food can also suffer from depression and low moods. Indeed the entire body will slow down. Often feeling tired and sleepy. You can even get a sense of a heavy weighed down feeling when your body is filled with excess fluids and phlegm.

To fix a cold and phlegm filled digestive system. Avoid consuming physically cold food and drink. Avoid phlegm producing foods like dairy. Then add heating foods, like small amounts of spices, alcohol, coffee or red or black teas. Slowly increase these amounts until the digestive system has warmed up and been brought back into the correct balance.

Now we can turn to heat in the intestines. There are two patterns involved. Let's start with heat and dryness. If you have eaten too much hot and drying foods or neglected to eat enough cooling, moistening and cleaning foods, then you may find your intestines starting to heat and dry their linings out. As soon as food enters from the stomach into these dried intestines, all the moisture is quickly pulled away from it. The dehydrated food has now shrunk in size and is having difficulty trying to slide its way through this dry intestine. As it travels through this really long tube, it gets even more dry and reduced in size, leaving you blocked up.

To fix this, you need to ingest good quality oils, like olive oil and oil from seeds. This helps to lubricate the lining of the intestine and helps food to slide through. You need to also increase your amount of cooling foods like vegetables. These will start to take heat and dryness away and remoisten the lining. Vegetable soups are quite useful for this purpose. Furthermore, you need to add bitter juices like grape, pomegranate and berries. These will cause fluids to build up directly in the intestine, moistening everything. They are often used in Chinese Medicine as natural laxatives. Try taking a half pint to a full pint a day for a few weeks and see the strong difference it makes.

Beware though, sometimes you can take too much bitter fluids in, causing them to purge the entire contents of the tube out. If this happens, you won't go to the toilet for a day or two, until the tube fills back up again.

Also if you have suffered badly from constipation, it is a good idea to start slowly to build up these cooling, moistening, purging foods. As the top of the intestine will be the first to be rectified, then the middle and finally the bottom. Foods will move quickly through the top moistened areas, which can lead to pile ups and traffic jams in the lower parts which can still be too dry. This produces cramps and pains. If this happens, gently massage your abdomen, and as the back log breaks up the cramps will disappear.

Fibre is commonly used in response to constipation in the West. This is not seen as a wise idea in the East. Fibre is a bulky food which cannot be properly digested. It passes through the digestive system and is excreted out intact. Unfortunately the body does not know fibre can't be broken down and wastes a massive amount of energy trying to digest it. This often does not resolve constipation but does lead to belly ache, bloating, tiredness and often large amounts of flatulence. Insoluble fibre as found in bran, brown rice and bread is far worse than the soluble fibre found in fruit etc., which dissolves in water to form a gel like substance.

Heat and dryness in the intestines can cause symptoms like odorous gas, cramps, pain, indigestion, dry small hard stools, piles or constipation. It can also cause the reduction of fluid and its nutrients in your blood. This can lead to anxiety, irritability, racing mind, anger and poor sleep. In the rest of the body, it can start to cause many of the other symptoms that we discussed in earlier chapters.

It does also cause a significant and dangerous problem with toxicity in the body. As rotten elements are not being removed through the colon. They are instead being absorbed as toxins into the system. This can produce many serious illnesses and also over burden the lungs, skin and bladder, the other organs which are involved in waste disposal.

The other pattern involving the intestine is heat, damp and phlegm. The food here is being overcooked as it passes through. This makes it rot and become putrid. Over time this will inflame, agitate, burn, destroy and mutate cells in the intestinal lining which may even lead to cancers. Heat causes movement, so you may often find sudden urges to defecate with this pattern. A classic sign of heat and toxins in the intestine, is that the bowel movement will have a strong and foul odour. Again you may have gas and indigestion that is quite rotten in smell. Your urine may also be a strong yellow and may smell.

This is a bad pattern to have, as fresh food is tainted as it enters this mix from the stomach. Because of this you will pull mostly poisons and toxins into your body. Which over time will heavily pollute it leading to most of our modern illnesses.

You need to completely clean up your diet. Immediately stop taking fats, greases, overly processed foods and other contaminants into your body. Also temporarily stop taking coffee, red and black tea, alcohol and spices. And add in lots of green tea, peppermint tea and bitter fruit and juices to reverse it.

Piles.

Piles can come from cold or from heat and damp. If from cold there is a lack of energy to hold blood strongly in the vessels causing them to bleed easily. With cold there won't be much pain. When heat is involved, it swells and expands the blood vessels, filling them with pressure and causing them to pop and bleed easily. If damp and phlegm are involved there will be even more inflammation in the blood vessels. These piles will be tender, swollen and painful. Avoid exerting and forcing yourself when using the toilet and treat the bigger pattern seen in the digestive tract to resolve and fix them.

Chapter Twenty Three   -   Fats And Oils.

Western dietary guidance has now finally started to emphasize the differences between fats. We have bad fats that raise dangerous cholesterol and block us up. And good ones that can help things move more freely and work more effectively in the body. This category should really be named bad fats and good oils. As this is a much clearer representation of their effects.

Bad fats usually come from animal fats and fats which have been processed and chemically altered such as hydrogenated oils and trans fats. Man made and altered fats should be avoided as much as possible. Our bodies are made from nature and have only natural means available to dissolve and cope with these fats. Quite often they fail to break them down, and instead allow them to accumulate and be the cause of many diseases.

The good helpful oils, generally come from plants such as olive oil and also from fish, nuts and seeds. When buying oils, try to find ones that have been cold pressed. These oils have been collected and bottled through cooler temperatures and the structures of the oil have been left purer and more intact.

Bad fats can cause considerable damage in the body. They congeal and thicken. Some may go off and turn into a sludge. Vessels will become filled by them, leading to a pressure that can cause breakages. This may result in strokes, clots and haemorrhages. Pressure can also cause aches and pains. It can put stress on organs as they try to push harder to do their jobs. This can cause them to wear and tire out more quickly. It can cause your energy levels to drop because of the increased work load. Bad fats can coat and pollute cells and cut off their supplies of nutrients and oxygen. They can lodge in your joints causing a type of arthritis. They can cause problems everywhere they come in contact with.

Good oils however, do the opposite. They help things slide and glide throughout the body. Organs can do their jobs more easily, conserving their energy and helping them last longer.

If you think of a car engine, if it has heavy thick blackened oil, this sludge can lodge in parts of it and clog them up. It can cause them to over work and wear out, or even break them from a build up of pressure. Good oil does the opposite, all parts of the engine become lubricated, move more effectively and last longer.

If we examine two areas in the body, the heart and the brain, we can easily see the effects of good oils and bad fats.

Fat can lodge in the blood vessels in the body. The heart still has to maintain the right levels of blood supply through these passageways. Because they are narrower, the heart has to push harder to get the right amount of blood supply around the body. Over time, under this pressure, it can weaken and wear out. There is also a chance of fat blocking one of the vessels in the heart itself, causing a heart attack. On the other hand if we have clean blood vessels and add a small amount of good fine oils. Then we find the movement of the heart can glide more easily. Conserving its energy and helping it last longer.

In the brain fats can gather and block up all the tiny connections. This can lead initially to poor memory, thought processing and concentration. And over time may eventually help to create illnesses like dementia. Whereas good oils actually help things move more easily and increase the speed of connections, which enhances your brain power.

It's not that difficult to switch over from fats to oils. Buy lean cuts of meat and trim away any fat from them. Use olive oil and other good ones when cooking. Switch from using butter on your bread and vegetables to drizzling olive oil over them. You can add any type of green herbs, like basil and oregano, to give oils more taste.

Fats are heavy, greasy and sticky and can easily accumulate in the body. Once they are in there, it is difficult to remove them. However, oils remain fluid like and do not gather so easily. The body can successfully clear away any excess of these. If you dip your finger in and out of butter. The butter will have formed lumps of itself on your finger. Dip it in and out of oil and you will be left with only a fine coating. So although they may contain the same number of calories, your body is far better able to process oil than it is to process thickened fats.

If you have heat and phlegm or toxins in your intestines, (foul odour from the bowel movement is the most telling sign). You must clean them before switching on to good oils. Otherwise you will just be mixing good oils in with bad greases. It would be like pouring fresh oil in on top of old thick black oil in your car engine. You need to take the sludge out of your intestines first, just like removing the old engine oil, before the good fresh stuff goes in. So cut back on all fats and oils in your diet. Add in bitter cleansing tastes like green tea, pomegranate, grapes and berries. Then after the odour goes, you can start to refill with good oils.

Chapter Twenty Four - How To Lose Weight.

There are many different diets in the West. Most of them are based around calorie restriction. This is not seen as a good idea in the East. As although you can lose weight by reducing calories, if you overdo it this will cause more long term harm than good. Apart from the immediate pressure you put on your body from having to keep things going without adequate fuel, you will start to eat into your Jing and hormones as well. This can weaken you and shorten your lifespan.

More directly, in terms of weight, you will weaken the very organs necessary to manage the successful breakdown and absorption of food. So when you come off your diet, those weakened organs will be unable to process foods at the same rates as before. Your now slowed metabolism will cause you to gain weight and get fat far more easily. I have come across many long term dieters, who have weakened their digestion and slowed their metabolism to such an extent, that they now live on children sized portions or even less. If they try to eat more than that, then weight piles on to them.

However, having said all that, if you do fall into the category of over eating, then you do need to cut back on calories to successfully lose weight.

Before we discuss the correct methods of dieting we will discuss bodily fat. There are two placements for fat inside the body. Its either pushed aside or its spread everywhere, including throughout all of the organs. The fat that has been pushed aside, to the other parts of your body is not so dangerous. Depending on your personal taste, you may not find it pretty, but it is not getting in the way or doing much damage. However, the fat in your blood vessels and organs is the real killer. It impedes things, leading to build ups that can rupture and cause heart attacks and strokes. It wastes your energy and can tire your organs, as they have to work harder, pushing and shoving things through all this fat. It can start to overheat and rot. Damaging cells around it, causing them to mutate.

Surprisingly, appearances can be very deceptive. Skinny people can actually be carrying lots of fat in their blood vessels and organs. Whereas some larger people, who gathered fat over years, but are now eating healthily, have excess fat built up on their outsides but have clear passageways through and around vessels and organs. These larger people will be much healthier and far less likely, than thin people with fatty deposits in organs, to get strokes, heart disease, diabetes and dementia etc.

When you diet and detoxify with bitter juices, green tea and so on. The first part of the body to be cleaned will be the organs and blood system. These are the parts the body is dependant on. After this, it will attend to more external areas of the body. Although you may remain fat for quite some time after changing your diet, your organs and more important insides will have cleaned themselves out. Within a couple of months you will feel and be healthier, happier and have far less of a chance of serious illnesses.

Now we come to the part that interests many people. The issue of losing weight. Weight gain can usually comes from two different patterns. The first involves a hot and toxic digestive system, and the second a weak cold digestive system. This can include a weak hormonal system as well.

Of course, sometimes people can get a mix of both. They may have both a hot polluted and a weak powerless digestive system. This is trickier to fix, but if you adopt a healthy diet, after some time the toxins will clear and then you can heat and power up your digestion to speed up the metabolism and lose weight.

Hot And Toxic Digestive System.

We will start with the hot and toxic digestive system. This is usually caused by consuming hot foods and rich phlegm creating ones. In this scenario, the rest of the body is likely to also display hot and toxic symptoms such as frustration, acne, anxiety, body odours, red face and so forth. The stomach when filled with fatty, gooey, hard to digest foods, starts to overheat, as it has retained them for too long. They clog and block it up. This causes it to remain dirty after use. This can lead to fresh food, even of good quality, being damaged as it is put into this already over heated and toxic stomach bag. All food now leaving the stomach and going into the intestines will be polluted and may not have been broken down properly. After time, the intestines too, will usually become clogged, dirty and putrid on the inside. Everything entering the digestive tract is now being tarnished. You will no longer get good quality energy and nutrients from your food but instead you will get lots of festering garbage building up in your system and making you fat.

To resolve this you need to stop putting in heating foods like coffee, alcohol and spices, in order to let your system cool down. Stop eating rich, phlegm filled foods like dairy, sugars, greases and fats. And finally flush your system clean. Use lots of green tea, bitter fruits and juices. Use mostly pomegranate, grapes and berries. And add some watered down lemon, lime or grapefruit juice. Rhubarb is also quite effective for clearing and cleaning the intestine. Finally add in some peppermint tea to cool, clean and create fast movement of food through the intestines.

Weak And Cold Digestive System.

The second pattern that creates weight gain is from weak digestion. Usually the body feels cold in this case. It may be lethargic, pale and weak. The mind may be depressed. The nose is often blocked or runny. There may be bloating and fluid retention. Often accompanied by loose or soft bowel movements without any odour. Other symptoms like indigestion and abdominal distension may also occur.

This pattern can come about from many different sources. It can come from consuming cold food and drinks, such as from salads or icy water with meals. And from other things like exposure to cold in winter. From weak hormones, chronic illness, accidents, sudden intense shocks or prolonged over work, study and stress. And cold and weak energy can even come from emotions like sadness, worry and depression. Basically from anything that slows and reduces energy levels in your body. When your energy becomes weak and depleted, there is insufficient power to break down and process foods. Which leads to a build up of fluid and undigested foods being pulled into the body and being pushed aside as unusable waste and fats.

The solution to this is quite easy and will not just burn up weight but will also make you feel stronger, more energetic and even more happy, as increased blood and energy supply will boost your brain. Firstly avoid rich damp forming foods like dairy. Obviously avoid fats, greases and sugars. Then make sure all foods and drinks entering the body are warm in temperature. Do not have anything cold. Temporarily reduce consumption of foods that are cold in nature, such as mineral filled vegetables and fruits like bananas and mangoes. And finally, slowly add small amounts of foods to your diet that are hot in nature and action. Such as alcohol, coffee, red and black tea. Spices are particularly good for the digestive system. Be careful not to add too many stimulants, as it can create too much heat and cause the system to swing too far to the hot side. So start with just one or two and slowly build up until you reach the right levels.

These stimulants will start to raise your metabolic rate, heating you up and drying away the fluids. The average body and brain burn 2,000 to 2,500 calories daily. If you speed up your metabolism and general activity levels in the body by 10 percent, you will burn up 200 to 250 extra calories. The equivalent of running for about 45 minutes. You can also physically warm up your abdomen and lower back, by wearing extra clothes and using heat pads and so forth.

Be warned, if you are already hot, don't further heat your body to lose weight. This could make you burn the weight quicker but can also congeal phlegm and fluids into harder nastier toxins which can lead to major illnesses like cancer, strokes and diabetes.

Exercise can be useful in reducing weight and in the appropriate ways can be beneficial to the body, (see the chapter on exercise). But I have always found in myself and in patients I have treated, that the right changes in diet has a far bigger and more long term impact on proper weight management and general health.

Chapter Twenty Five   -   Cravings And Appetite.

In this chapter we will discuss cravings. It is an important issue, not just in terms of people trying to lose weight, where cravings can build up so intensely, that they make you binge and fall off the diet. But also it is a good indicator as to whether or not you are missing some vital ingredients from your diet. If you have a well balanced diet, you will not have any cravings.

Cravings can come about as the brain is checking for levels of nutrients in the blood stream. If something is missing or levels are low, the brain increases your appetite and causes an urge to eat some type of food containing the needed ingredient. The desire will come in whatever form it is used to consuming which contains that missing element in it. For example, when energy is low, the most common craving Westerners get will be in the form of sugar. This may be cakes, sweets, sugary drinks and so forth.

To get around cravings we must replace bad foods with good foods. If we just go without the food, then cravings will increase until they become intolerable. People's diets usually crash because they have starved their bodies until the cravings are too intense. Most commonly people miss energy when they are on a diet, hence the desire for sugary high energy foods. We can replace these with white rice, which is excellent for producing a good constant stream of energy. And if you are in a cold pattern, the addition of small amounts of spices and alcohol will also raise your energy levels.

At the start, when you move away from toxic foods the brain is a little lost. It takes a few weeks or even several months in some people, for it to adjust to new foods. Once it has, you will be surprised by the changes that take place. You will find that you start to want these new healthier foods and you will naturally begin to lose desire for the older more unhealthy ones you used to like.

Initially I struggled when I switched to good foods, but after a while, I started to lose interest in sugar and chocolate and so on. My body began to reject these foods all by itself. And if from old habits, I decided to have a so called treat, instead of feeling good from it, I would feel blocked up and sickly. You will eventually find this too. That your body as it fills up with good healthy nutrients and clean energy, no longer wants junk foods and it naturally puts you off them.

Good healthy foods that are excellent at beating cravings and reducing appetite are white rice for general energy. A little coffee, alcohol or spices with food if you are feeling cold, sluggish and tired. And for general nutrients and body care you need vegetables, eggs, seeds and nuts.

Chapter Twenty Six - General Healthy Eating And More Weight Loss Tips.

1) Keep a food diary. Write down everything you are eating and drinking throughout each day. Quite often when people can actually see how much junk there can be in their diet, it is enough to put them off it. Many people are surprised how a little treat here and there, suddenly amounts to a lot of potentially harmful toxins and phlegm creating substances over a week. By keeping a diary for a few weeks, you can better manage your diet. You can reflect on and clearly sees what needs to be reduced, increased or altered, to produce more effective and efficient results.

2) Read the labels on all packaging. Get used to seeing exactly what chemicals and extras are being added. Check for things ending in "ose". Such as glucose, lactose and sucrose. They are all types of sugar. Try to find the most natural foods. The ones with the least amount of additives, preservatives, artificial colourings and flavourings. Avoid trans fats and hydrogenated fat. These are cheap chemically altered vegetable fats used to bulk up foods and to preserve them. They have no nutritional value but do cause levels of bad cholesterol to rise. Many chemical preservatives don't just stop nature from rotting and breaking down foods, but as we are also part of nature and use similar processes as it, they can stop us from being able to digest them as well. This can lead to dangerous and destructive chemicals building up in our systems.

Artificial colours and chemicals used to colour our food and drink have been linked to cancer (studies in rats have indicated this), asthma and more recently to hyperactivity in children. A major British study in the Lancet reported that artificial colourings and preservatives did increase hyperactivity in children. This led to the European Food Standards Agency to recommend that companies voluntarily remove them from their products.

Check the ingredients on the back of the product match what the item is actually supposed to be. Quite often some fruit juices are advertised as berry but when you read the label, it might say 20 percent berry, 70 percent apple and 10 percent banana. This will create different flavours and cause the juice to act in a different way. Also check for things like added sugars. If the sugar is from the fruit itself, then this is fine. But for most fruit juices you don't want any other sugars added to them. The exception is probably cranberry juice. As it is intensely bitter, it is very hard to find it without any added sugar. In this case the extreme bitter taste will push the sticky sugar away from the cells and won't harm the body, so it is ok.

3) Check the calorie levels on the labels too. You might be shocked like I was, to find that one small cake may have as much as 500 or 600 calories in it. You could have more than a whole plate of rice and vegetables for that. Most junk foods have high calorie counts and low nutrient levels. If the brain is not getting all the nutrients it requires, it will cause cravings for more food and you will start to overeat. It will also not have enough power to support functions like thought processing, memory and concentration. Your mood too may drop and you could find yourself in low spirits or even depressed. A plate of vegetables and rice will provide all your nutrients through the vegetables and energy through the rice. This will satisfy your hunger and stop cravings and feed your mind all it needs to keep it active, healthy and happy.

Surprisingly, many overweight people are deficient in a lot of vitamins and minerals. Although they have a high calorie intake, many of these foods contain just nutritionally deficient empty calories, which pile on weight but leave the body undernourished and the brain unsupported and still hungry. Many processed foods are no longer useful at all. Compare the taste of freshly squeezed orange juice with many concentrated versions. They are not even close in taste. When food is over processed it can become just dead useless calories.

A team at the University College Of London found that there was a 58 percent higher risk of depression when you compared those who ate the most processed foods to those who ate the least, in their study of 3,500 participants. As reported in the Journal of Psychiatry.

4) If you have a setback and eat something bad, don't feel guilty. This will just use your energy up and upset your mind. That will make you want to crave even more energy from food. Just write it off. Forget about it. And move on as quickly as possible, re-focusing your mind on the goals and healthy new system that you do want to achieve.

Everyone has bad days and makes mistakes. Any new change in your life will take time to accomplish. But all that is really needed is practice and perseverance. As long as you don't give up, it will eventually become a natural part of you, that takes no effort to maintain.

5) Don't over eat. Try not to fill your stomach at each meal. This sounds so obvious but has become quite a common habit for most people. So eat consciously and become aware of it. If your stomach is too full at the end of a meal, then it cannot churn and mix enzymes effectively, leading to decreased ability to fully breakdown foods. This can easily make you fat, tired and sick. An easy way to avoid this, is to simply use smaller plates for meals.

6) When shopping avoid the aisles that have unhealthy foods in them. When they are out of sight and out of mind, you will be far less tempted. Avoid too, having junk food in your home. Don't use the excuse that it is only there for guests. If you know its there your mind will think and dwell on it, and often give in to that temptation.

Make a firm commitment to your subconscious right now, that you are leaving behind all foods that make you ill. And are now embracing those that will increase your health, vitality and your real happiness.

7) If you feel your energy system start to drop, eat something like rice. Don't wait until you are really hungry or you will over eat. If you feel really low have a small amount of coffee, spices or alcohol with your food. This will quickly revive your energy and will power. But don't do this too often if you are affected by heat patterns as you can make them worse.

Avoid over working or over studying. Anything that will really deplete you. Try to be more consistent and moderate in your actions so you can keep energy levels high.

When you are dieting, be sure to eat small quantities of very rich foods, such as nuts, seeds, seaweed and eggs. These are jam packed with nutrients. Your brain checks for nutrients all the time in your blood stream, if it's missing some it will send cravings out for food. By eating these densely packed nutritious foods, you will keep levels of essential ingredients high in the body and brain. This will stop cravings and dramatically lower hunger levels.

8) Get good rest and sleep. If you miss sleep your body won't have enough energy the next day. So it won't be able to run effectively and will create more cravings for extra food to gain power to offset this. The cravings are more likely to be for a quick source of energy such as sugary and fatty foods. This may lead to weight gain and will pollute your body at the same time.

9) Avoid artificial sweeteners and diet foods. Studies have shown that although low in calories, these still cause weight gain. Anything with a sweet taste is still sticky. It can still bind and trap things into the body. Regardless of its number of calories. They are also not producing the energy the body requires, so the mind will keep craving more until it has been satisfied.

Research by a team at the University of Alberta, published in the journal Obesity, showed that when young rats were fed low calorie versions of foods they would start to overeat. Another study by scientists at Purdue University published in the journal Behavioural Neuroscience, found similar results. That rats fed saccharin ended up eating more calories, putting on more fat and gaining more weight than rats who were fed ordinary sugar instead of the artificial sweetener. This was again backed up by similar findings from Duke University, published in the journal Of Toxicology And Environmental Health.

10) Eat slowly or you will overeat. Your mouth can consume food far faster than your stomach can break it down. The brain can't tell if you have had enough food until it starts to pick up these nutrients in the blood stream. So you need to eat slow enough, to allow the breakdown process to occur, and the brain to then shut your hunger and desire for food off.

11) Learn and practice breathing and Qi Gong exercises. Full details are given later. For the moment, all you need to know is that it will bring clarity to your mind and strengthen your ability to choose what you are doing rather than being led by impulses. It will also boost your energy, speed up your metabolism and generally lower your need and desire for high energy unhealthy foods like sugars and bad fats. If you have lots of energy already from breathing properly and Qi Gong, then you don't need so much at all from your food. This is similar to what happens to many people in summer. They are getting plenty of extra energy from the sun and so find that they lose their appetite for food.

12) Beware of some of the new so called health foods. Many of them have taken an extract from a good healthy food source and simply added it into their product. Then they claim that their product is some sort of super food providing this or that in the body. This is completely misleading. It's like sweeping dirt under your carpet. The original product is still as bad as ever. As soon as you mix a healthy food with an unhealthy one, you will tarnish its properties and it will not give the same effect. The best way to get that other genuinely good ingredient is through a healthy diet.

Low fat foods are often misleading. Many actually only imply reduced levels of fat in comparison to the original product. For example, butter has one of the highest levels of fat per gram compared to the vast majority of other foods. Low fat butter has some of this removed but is still high in fat compared to most other foods. So always read the ingredients, calorie counts and other information even on the labels of low fat foods.

13) When eating out or buying processed foods, always go for the healthiest options you can find. This won't just help you, but will encourage businesses to start producing healthier foods. They will have to come up with new and better options once there is a market for them. At the moment the food industry is taking advantage of us, by chemically altering our foods and using the cheapest means of mass producing them. But as consumers, we have the power and the responsibility to lead industry to higher standards. We just need to exercise our buying power in the right directions to more healthy and nutritious food. Buy organic and more natural less interfered with foods, as often as you can. Send them a clear message of the high quality we want and expect from our foods.

Processed meats like bacon and ham, now often contain inorganic phosphate salts. A common additive used to retain fluids and bulk up meats to increase their price. This has been strongly linked to fuelling the growth of tumours and cancers in laboratory studies.

Evidence gathered by the World Cancer Research Fund suggests that eating 150 grams of processed meats, such as beef and ham, increases your chances of bowel cancer by 63 percent.

In a study of 190,545 people by a team at the University of Hawaii. It was noted that people who ate the most processed meat had a 67 percent higher chance of developing pancreatic cancer than those who ate the least.

Research at the Karolinska Institute concluded that of 61,433 women in their study, those who ate the most cured meats, such as bacon, sausages and smoked meats, doubled their risk of stomach cancer.

14) Bribe your children to eat well. Promise them a day out or a gift if they eat some new vegetables daily for a month or two. If they manage to eat it for that time they will grow used to it, their taste buds will alter and most will leave it in their diets for good thereafter.

But don't force good foods on them, as it will cause their subconscious to connect healthy foods with punishment and bad experiences. And this may put them off these foods for many years.

By giving them a good start with diet, you are setting them up for a healthy positive bright future.

15) Start growing your own fruit and vegetables. There are many natural alternatives you can use instead of the harsh and unsafe pesticides and chemicals used in modern farming methods of mass production. The food will also have a stronger flavour and taste better.

Other benefits include that you will get out into the sun and fresh air more. You will get good exercise, be able to socialize and swap ideas with fellow enthusiasts. You can teach your children about growing healthy food and have more family time with them. And you will save yourself money on the cost of store bought fruit and vegetables.

16) Keep a good straight posture after eating meals. If you sit hunched up, working at a desk after lunch or breakfast, you will physically squash your stomach and intestines. This prevents them from breaking food down successfully. And instead causes it to stagnate and let out gasses, leading to cramps and indigestion. If you suffer from this, drink peppermint tea with and after meals. Take a rest from work after eating or go for a gentle stroll to help things move through your intestines.

17) Reduce the amount of water you consume. There was an incorrect notion circulated in the West not so long ago, that people should drink at least eight large glasses of water a day. That this would detoxify them and make them more healthy. Well simply, it doesn't. What it does do is put a tremendous strain on your body to have to deal with all that excess fluid. It wastes your energy and your resources. It can overcool your system, particularly the digestion, slowing down your metabolism, damaging and weakening your kidneys and the production of hormones. It can encourage weight gain and help you to retain unwanted fluids. Yes, you should definitely have fluid when you are thirsty and in general a glass or two of plain water a day. But the majority of your fluids should come through vegetables, green tea, peppermint tea, fruit juices and other foods. As we are now aware, if we want to detox, then fluids or foods that taste bitter are our best options.

18) Generally you need to change your diet according to the season and climate. Foods growing in certain climates have adapted to them and evolved over thousands and thousands of years. For example, bananas grow in very hot and dry climates. They have a sweet taste and lots of minerals in them to keep them moist and cool. As soon as you chew one, your mouth becomes very wet and sticky. On the other hand, we have watercress. It is peppery and grows in watery areas, such as by rivers and marshes. Its spicy zest expectorates fluids and stops the watercress become overwhelmed and turning into mush. Another example is cacti, A cactus grows in hot dry desserts, so it has developed moistening and cooling properties to balance itself against this.

If you live in a damp wet climate like Ireland. You should avoid eating bananas, especially in winter. They will create phlegm and over cool and weaken your digestion. You need a very strong digestive system to break them down. Banana plants would not grow or fruit properly in Ireland. They would rot from the rain, cold and damp.

In general eat more cooling foods in summer. And more warming foods in winter. However because we now have air conditioning and central heating systems, this traditional advice has become somewhat distorted. So be aware of it, but always pay attention to the higher rule of balancing whatever is existing in your personal bodily system.

19) Try to eat in a calm, relaxed and peaceful state. Allow time for your digestion to work after having a meal. Avoid working, studying, reading arguing, rushing or any excessive strong emotional states. All these activities and states rob energy that your digestive system needs to break food down. They will slow your metabolism down and can cause many other problems such as bloating, gas and pains etc.

20) Use natural raw cane sugar or honey as a sweetener if required. A healthy body, usually does not crave sugar when it has good supplies of energy. But if your brain has been used to consuming it, then these will help you wean yourself away from more processed man made sugars. Eventually you should be able to give up sugar entirely, unless you are using it to medicinally balance your body. When you are eating the right foods and using others methods like proper breathing and Qi Gong, to gather energy, you should find you need less and less sugar.

21) Different types of cooking can affect the qualities in your food. When you boil or steam food, it generally weakens it. Giving hot natured food, like spices, cooler properties. When you boil onions, you will notice it causes them to lose their aroma and sting. The longer you boil, the weaker things become, so avoid boiling for too long.

Also sometimes you could avoid discarding the water you used for boiling. As this is filled with lots of nutrients from the food. A way to do this is through soups and stews.

A soup or stew can be quite beneficial, as it helps to soften and pre-digest the food. Soups and stews can be used to build up weak constitutions and for those trying to regain strength after and during illness.

When you cook with oils, such as roasting and frying. The oils bind to the food, sealing them and locking in flavours, nutrients and energy. This generally increases the heating nature of the food and makes it more active. You should cook foods thoroughly but quickly when frying. Obviously avoid burning and over crisping your foods. As this damaged food cannot be digested and has been linked in modern studies to cancer.

22) The next tip is very important for general health and also for losing weight. You should completely reverse the Western way of having a small breakfast (or even skipping it, as some people do). Having a medium sized lunch and finishing with a big dinner. This modern way of eating is completely wrong. Asians eat their meals in the opposite proportions. Big breakfast, medium lunch, and small evening meal. Even older generations in the West ate their meals like this. There is an old Western saying, "Breakfast like a king, lunch like a prince and dinner like a pauper".

This is very important to do. And is one of the best things to do to lose weight, you can eat the same amount of calories as you would normally do. But in the reverse order. You should find that you start to lose weight from this alone. Western study after study is now proving this theory right. That this is the correct way of eating.

Logic and common sense also tells you this is the correct way of eating. You need energy from a big meal to keep you going all day long. At night you don't need a big belly full of food to help you to sleep. We have evolved in this form for over the last 80,000 plus years. In those times, we would rise early at dawn, get up, hunt and gather food and then eat it. In winter, it could get dark as early as four pm. People did not eat late at night. Our digestive systems are designed to be strong and have energy in the early hours of the day. At night they are not needed during sleep, so the body has evolved to remove energy from them and pass it to the other organs which are involved with sleep.

It comes down to this. If you eat at night, your digestion has insufficient power to break down the food properly. It will leave partially digested food in your intestines and stomach. Damaging them and blocking and bloating you. This may cause it to pull harmful fats and phlegm into the body. Leaving you only partially nourished and also gaining excessive weight. If you want to lose weight, have a big breakfast, medium lunch and small meal before five pm. Avoid eating after this time.

Many Western studies are now beginning to back up this way of eating. A study from a team at the University of Minnesota, reported in the journal Paediatrics, found that teenagers who skipped breakfast were on average five pounds heavier than those who did not.

A study in the journal Obesity by researchers at Northwestern University noted that when mice were fed at unusual times, when they would normally be asleep. They put on 48 percent more weight over six weeks than those who were fed at their normal eating times.

A study by Dr. Jakubowicz from Virginia Commonwealth University found that dieters who followed the big breakfast, medium lunch and small dinner model, lost on average four times as much as the group who ate in the existing Western way.

Researchers at Harvard Medical School also found that people who ate breakfast were a third less likely to be obese.

23) Try to learn from your body every time you eat something. Try to feel and see what effects it is having on you. What it does in your digestive tract. Is it sitting there like a lump in your belly. Has it caused bloating, gas and cramps. Were you constipated or was your bowel movement loose or odorous later on, or the next day. And also reflect on what has happened in the rest of you. Did you heat up or cool down. Get a high followed by a low. Feel good strong energy or feel tired. Feel sweaty or thirsty. Feel anxious or relaxed and so forth. Try to start matching foods with their effects. Over time you will become a master of this and clearly be able to see what they are doing to you.

Beware of stimulants like coffee, alcohol and spice. They can make you feel pretty good when you take them. But if you start to take too much, they will do the opposite. They will give you a dead energy with a tired and drained feeling at the same time.

One way of understanding foods, is to try and imagine how they will react on the living tissue of your hand. Whether they will cause heat, cold, stickiness or dryness etc. For example, if you were to think of porridge and honey on your hand, you would see it as very sticky and gooey. It will do the same in your intestine and may overheat it and block it up. A better combination would be porridge and bitter berries or grapes. You can even try adding fruit juice to your porridge to cool it down. This would cause more movement on your hand and through your stomach, as the living tissues and cells react and pull away from the bitter taste.

Chapter Twenty Seven   -   Reprogram Your Mind.

As we grow up as children, our brains are like sponges. They absorb and are easily influenced by so much around us. Often they are given the wrong messages and ideas. Once these have been implanted in our subconscious minds, they take on a life of their own. We can be stuck with these incorrect ideas for many many years. Unfortunately, some people never wake up. They never start to think for themselves. They instead continue, like robots, to spew out the same old misguided beliefs they learnt as a child. The outcome of this is that they end up living in a very ignorant and blind world.

In regard to food, it is very important that we correct these erroneous ideas which were pushed into our subconscious. We need to completely alter what our minds see as happy foods and see as unpleasant ones. It all begins with things like birthday parties, where the main event is a rich creamy spongy chocolate cake or such like, accompanied by fizzy sugary drinks, sweets and crisps. What this is doing to your brain is implanting the idea that happiness is associated with junk food. That junk food is special and a treat. That from now on, every time you feel low, you don't have to deal with and fix your problems, but instead can rely on this junk for comfort. Problem is, it produces only fleeting pleasure and leaves you filled with toxins and in a worse place than from where you started at.

When we think about it logically we should be put off gooey, greasy, sticky, tarry, blackened fry ups and burgers and the like. We certainly wouldn't want to bathe in or rub that stuff into our skin as a moisturiser. Yet our minds have been influenced to accept that this food is appealing and is a treat. Everything in life is to do with perspective. You are trapped until you start to think for yourself and break free to see things for what they really are. In the West, we happily eat cows and are appalled if we hear of Asians eating dogs. However in many Indian religions, cows are sacred animals. And they are appalled to hear of us eating them. In Africa many tribes would eat insects for protein, some Westerners would be sickened by the idea of this, without realising that many of their favourite foods coloured red contain the crushed Cochineal beetle and its eggs. It is even in most red lipsticks commonly used by women. Everything is just perspective. What has been put into your mind by others and what they have conned you into believing. Modern advertising has a field day with this. It links strong emotions of happy events with foods to subconsciously link them in your mind. They would have us believe that by drinking certain soft drinks you will be more popular and cool. Even chocolate is now promoted as being sexy and orgasmic. We need to stop listening to others and start thinking for ourselves.

To reprogram our minds, all we need to do is to wake up. To start to form our own independent judgements. To see things for what they truly are. From this new awareness, intelligence and acceptance of this real truth, we can start to rewrite the incorrect stored logic in our subconscious. To do this, we need to repetitively inform it of what we now really want. It is quite easy to do. But it does take focus and patience. You need to repeat your new desire in a concentrated way several times a day to your subconscious. This may take weeks or even months of repetition, before it over writes the old belief with this new one. You will learn more about this important and useful skill of influencing and changing your subconscious in later chapters.

So start to change your views of foods. See the bad ones for what they really are. Fatty, greasy, gooey, slimy, snotty, sticky and putrid. Start to associate them in your mind with disease. Imagine them blocking you up and rotting in your organs and body. Imagine them sitting in your brain, gluing it up and starting to form dementia. Imagine your heart starting to splutter and choke up from all that grease and fat gathering in your arteries.

Now imagine the opposite. How all that shiny fresh vegetables and fruit, those lean strips of chicken and fish, those glossy natural oils, nuts and seeds, will build strong clean cells and nourish you. Providing you with every element you need to remain powerful, vibrant, young, fit and healthy.

If you are eating food for comfort, it is essential to learn how to replace this habit with more positive ones. Later we will discuss methods of dealing with stress and learning how to create and bring happiness into your life.

If you have kids, break the mould and don't start to form bad habits in their minds. Avoid causing future suffering and problems for them, by rewarding them with love, pleasant and kind words and praise, rather than with sweets and treats.

When having guests over for celebrations and socializing, try to base it on events other than food or at least make it very healthy food. Don't be afraid to go against the grain and tell people what you are up to. Let them know you are trying to improve your health and theirs. Many people are a little overwhelmed by the different view of life in Chinese Medicine and in Asia. But once they start to see the profound logic and commonsense in it, they become quickly interested in it and want to know much more. It becomes a very lively topic of conversation.

One of the problems, we have in the West these days, is that we don't spend anytime preparing or being creative with our food. Healthy foods are not boring. Both Chinese and Indian cultures have an amazing variety of delicious healthy meals. However, the food you get in some Chinese and Indian restaurants is misguiding and quite unlike the real stuff you find in Asia. It has been marketed towards the tastes of Westerners and can be overly spicy and filled with fats and so on.

For tasty choices, we just need to start reading recipe books and experimenting. Shop in Asian supermarkets to get more variety in your diet. Expand your knowledge and selection of foods to keep things interesting. Don't be afraid to ask the shop assistants plenty of questions. Most will be happy to help you and get the extra business.

We can spend more time in the kitchen or even join cookery classes. It might become a very interesting hobby. You may even meet new friends and interesting people. You don't have to stick with tradition either. Feel free to make up your own meals. Traditions change and cultures change with each different passing generation. What's cool in one part of the world is not cool in another. So break free from all that nonsense and mental imprisonment. Experiment and find out what you like and go with that. If you want, even put a sprinkle of spices on a fruit salad. As unusual as this sounds, it is actually a good combination. Hot spices balanced with cooling fruits.

So get creative. And do more inventive home cooking, it is generally the best and healthiest as you are completely in charge of allowing whatever ingredients go into it.

Chapter Twenty Eight - Common Foods And Their Actions.

In this chapter we will discuss some everyday foods and describe the effects they have on the body. Do remember as foods ripen and age their tastes will change and with that their actions also become different. Generally the more intense the flavour and the odour, then the more exaggerated the action will be in the body.

Let's Start With Some Very Important Foods.

Rice.

White rice is a great food. It is a major source, perhaps the best, of good healthy food energy. In the West, people mistakenly throw white rice in with other highly processed white foods like bread. They claim that it too has as equally unhealthy properties as these others. But this is not the case at all. White rice is still basically the same on the inside as brown rice. It has just had minor adjustments, such as the outer fibrous husk being removed and then the grain being polished.

The Chinese character for energy "Qi", is made up of symbols for rice and air. Rice simply provides great energy for the entire body, mind and spirit. It is a huge part of most Asian diets. With some people consuming it as much as four times a day. Breakfast, lunch and dinner and then also even as snacks and sweets in-between. You can mix rice with most meals. You can turn it into healthy porridges and soups. It is a wonderful base food.

Now you are probably wondering why I keep mentioning white rice instead of brown rice, which is viewed as healthier in the West. Well on paper, it definitely is healthier. It has far more vitamins, minerals and nutrients in it. The problem however is all the fibre that it also contains. After most people, particularly those with weak digestive systems, eat brown rice, they often end up feeling bloated, tired and gassy. This is because the fibre cannot be digested. The body continually tries to break it down, but then quite often runs out of energy, leaving the remains to sit in and obstruct your intestines. It ferments and turns turbid making you feel unwell. On top of that, if you have had vegetables with your brown rice, there is no power to digest them, which means you will be deprived of their nutrients too. However, with white rice we see a completely different picture. It starts to break down easily, releasing its energy as it does so. This energy helps to power up the intestines and digestion, giving them more ability to digest all the vegetables that accompanied the white rice.

Vegetables have a far greater amount of nutrients than white or brown rice. So anything that aids their digestion, in this case the white rice, is very valuable. Overall the combination of the white rice and vegetables, when put through the process of human digestion, will end up giving your body more energy and nutrients, than the combination of brown rice and vegetables would do.

Vegetables.

Now vegetables have different flavours and do different things. But in general they provide the heavier elements that cool and preserve the body. They build the yin, cooling, nourishing, moistening side of the body. Most vegetables are cold in nature, with the exception of peppers, chilli, onions and spicy tasting vegetables, which create movement, heat and usually expectorate.

It is a good idea, if you have a clean diet and are not filled with phlegm and toxins to include a little spice when you are eating them. This will add extra power to your digestion, to more successfully break them down and absorb all their cooling minerals and nutrients.

They also provide a lot of the essential building materials to regenerate our cells and bodies. Just like other foods, depending on their weight, density and strength of flavour, they will break down in different areas of the body and create their effects there. So it is always good advice to get a selection of them to cater for everywhere in the body.

Plants are natural and water based. So it is easier for the body to obtain nutrients from them, than from meat products or processed foods. Their high levels of nutrients are more accessible and easily assimilated into the body.

Vegetable fats are also very different to animal fats. They are mostly unsaturated fats which have a good effect to lubricate and help free movement inside us. Unlike animal fats which can clog us up.

There is a strong science starting to develop in the West that confirms what Asians have known for thousands of years. Rice and vegetable based diets with small portions of animal products, once or twice a week, will keep you healthy, prevent most diseases and increase your longevity. The traditional Chinese diet includes exactly that. Lots of rice, vegetables and infrequent amounts of meat. Perhaps just once a week or less.

The Japanese too eat very little meat. Instead they prefer fish. In Japan in the seventh century, a famous Buddhist emperor banned the consumption of all land animals. Leaving only fish to be eaten. The law lasted over twelve hundred years until 1873. Not only did the cows, sheep, pigs and other animals have a good time from this ban, but the net result was to create a very healthy population. Even today in Japan, all rates of diseases, such as heart disease, cancer and so forth, are still much lower than in America. They have more centenarians, people over the age of one hundred years, per head of population than anywhere else in the developed world. Even the popular Mediterranean diet, promoted as very healthy and life prolonging in the West, also has only limited portions of meat and dairy in it.

A study published in the British Journal of Cancer found that vegetarians were 12 percent less likely to develop cancer than their meat eating counter parts. This went up to 45 percent for some cancers such as leukaemia, stomach cancer and bladder cancer.

A team at the University of California found that eating 5 to 9 portions of fruit and vegetables daily reduce the risk of pancreatic cancer by 50 percent. As reported in Cancer, Epidemiology, Biomarkers and Prevention Journal.

Research by scientists at Georgetown University showed that chemicals in vegetables like broccoli, cabbage and cauliflower boost DNA repair in cells which may stop them becoming cancerous, as reported in the British Journal Of Cancer.

There are other reasons to increase vegetables and reduce meat intake Firstly it is good for the environment. Cows and sheep produce methane gas. This is much more damaging than carbon dioxide. They also give us manure, heavy in nitrates which pollute our water and air. The United Nations Food And Agriculture Organisation has reported that this warms our planet even more than pollution from transport. On top of all that, cows and sheep eat about eight kilos of grains for every one kilo of meat they produce. This is obviously a very inefficient use of our food supplies. In a separate report in 2009, the United Nations Food And Agriculture Organisation issued a statement, saying there are now over one billion people suffering from hunger in the world, that's one sixth of the world's population. If we all ate less meat. We would be helping ourselves get and stay healthier. Helping the planet by polluting it less. Helping to leave enough food for everyone and reducing prices of food in poorer nations. And of course, I am sure lots of animals would be happier too.

Mushrooms have special qualities in Chinese Medicine. They are linked to boosting energy for hormones and the immune system. Reishi and Shitake mushrooms are particularly useful. But most types will still help create energy for the production of hormones.

A study from a team at the University of Western Australia, found that women who ate 10 grams of fresh mushrooms daily were 64 percent less likely to develop breast cancer. Women who combined mushrooms and green tea saw their risk reduced by almost 90 percent.

The top two recommendations by the American Cancer Society are to choose most of the foods you eat from plant sources and to limit your intake of high fat foods, particularly from animal sources.

One final thing to discuss in this section is sea vegetables. There are many types of seaweed we can buy in our main supermarkets and in Asian stores. We can also supplement our diet with kelp and spirulina tablets. Spirulina contains all the essential amino acids and is a very rich source of minerals. Sea vegetables are a fantastic source of nutrients. For example, the common types of sea weed found in sushi rolls have as much as twelve times the amount of calcium in them per gram compared with cow's milk. In Chinese Medicine they can be used to cool and nourish the body, in particular providing nutrients for the liver, kidneys and hormones. Seaweed can be cut into strips and used in soups, salads, snacks and sushi.

We leave this passage with an interesting quote from Albert Einstein. "Nothing will benefit human health and increase chances for survival on earth as much as evolution to a vegetarian diet". In his time, Einstein, one of the greatest scientists the world has ever known, had figured out how important it is to maximize intake of plants and reduce intake of meats.

Dairy.

It is rare that the Chinese will avoid any type of food. They will usually and quite happily even eat insects and other types of animals we wouldn't even consider touching in the West. However, the exception is dairy. In Chinese Medicine, dairy is considered as being far too rich. It creates phlegm. And lots and lots of it. This phlegm commonly collects in the body as fat. And in the lungs and nose as mucus.

When the lungs are blocked and not functioning fully, you will not get enough oxygen and energy through them into your blood and you will become tired. In particular, your immune system will weaken, leaving you more vulnerable to infections. This will cause substantially more colds and flu in winter. These will also tend to be more prolonged and drawn out. And will produce more intense symptoms. It can also, by blocking and weakening digestion, prevent the rest of your food from being properly absorbed into the body.

Milk has several problems. For starters, it has very high levels of fat. Then there is lactose, a type of sugar. Most people in the world are lactose intolerant and cannot break it down. It also contains casein which is bonded with calcium and is very difficult to digest. Casein is actually used as a base in wood glue.

Milk is sold to us under the guise that it is essential for our bones. This is ridiculous when you consider that the Chinese, who won't drink milk, have some of the lowest rates of osteoporosis, that is brittle bones disease, in the entire world. Far less than the biggest milk drinkers in the West, the Americans and the Europeans. Calcium can be found in many parts of people's diets, particularly in green leafy vegetables, which contain it in a much more usable and extractable form. Incidentally, cows get their calcium from eating foods like green grass. Soya is also another great provider of calcium. With soya milk, gram for gram, nearly matching the calcium level of cow's milk. Milk and its associated products, cheese, cream, butter, ice cream and yoghurts have all been linked to many illnesses in modern Western scientific studies. In Chinese Medicine, if you suffer from phlegm in any form in the body, you should change over immediately to a milk substitute. Particularly if you are overweight or have digestive problems, allergies, lung problems and nasal and sinus problems.

Long term if milk is overheated in the body, Chinese Medicine would associate it with toxic phlegm which may cause heart disease, strokes, cancers, tumours, and cysts throughout the body. It is also commonly associated with blocking up the circulation in the mind, giving poor concentration and memory. Over time this may lead to Alzheimer's disease and dementia.

There are many alternatives these days. Rice milk, which is very low in fat and is energy giving. Soya milk, again low in calories, and provides the same levels of nutrients and proteins as regular cow's milk. And even goat's milk. Goat's milk is easier to digest than cow's milk. They are smaller animals and like us have only one stomach.

Cows actually have four compartments that act like stomachs. This allows them to really digest and breakdown foods. Their calves are ideally set up to drink their mothers' milk. Unfortunately we are not. So unless we are starving and there is nothing else around, the healthier option is to pass on milk and its related products.

A study by researchers at the Washington University School Of Medicine for the National Institutes Of Health found that a 69 percent decrease in crying and 25 percent decrease in discomfort from colic, occurred when babies were taken off cow's milk formula.

The Physicians' Health Study of 20,885 doctors, noted that men who drank two and a half servings of dairy were 30 percent more likely to suffer prostate cancer than those who had less than half a serving daily. The Health Professionals Follow-up study concluded that men who had high levels of dairy in their diet had 70 percent more chance of prostate cancer.

There have been numerous studies linking an increased rate of breast cancer with dairy consumption. Reports in Cancer Research, Journal of the National Cancer Institute and the British Journal Of Cancer all showed higher correlations of breast cancer as levels of dairy increased in women's diets.

In the International Journal Of Cardiology, scientists who studied seven countries found that heart disease deaths rose as milk consumption rose. Studies reported in The Lancet and the Journal Of Internal Medicine both concluded that fats and proteins from dairy both strongly increased deaths from heart disease.

Researchers from Yale University found that after examining 34 different studies, countries like the U.S.A, Sweden and Finland, the highest consumers of meat and dairy, also had the highest rates of osteoporosis.

A study published in the Annals Of Allergy by a team at Georgetown University noted up to 86 percent of ear infections in children improved when they stopped taking milk and other allergens.

Researchers at the Karolinska Institute reported in the American Journal Of Clinical Nutrition that women who had four servings of dairy per day had twice the risk of serious ovarian cancer than those who had fewer than two servings.

Fruits.

Fruit can generally be sweet, sour, bitter or a combination of them. Remember to taste them, in order to figure out their actions. For example, red grapes can be very bitter and cleansing or then can be sweet with subtle bitter undertones which will give them active properties of energizing and gently cleaning.

Some other common fruits are listed below.

Pomegranate - Usually bitter tasting. It is a great all round cleanser. Pomegranates can be messy to eat, so quite often it is easier to take them in a juice form. You should have at least five of them a week. In Western terms, pomegranates have been found to have nearly every type of anti-oxidants. Anti-oxidants are believed to mop up and deal with disease causing free radicals in the body.

Cranberry - Bitter tasting. It is very useful for cleansing the kidneys and the bladder.

Blueberries, raspberries, plums, prunes and cherries - Bitter and / or sour tasting. They are all good cleansers.
Rhubarb - Bitter in taste. It is a good cleanser. Particularly for the lower body and the colon.

Grapefruit, lemon and lime - Very bitter in taste. They are all very strong cleansers and can weaken the body if overused. Keep these for occasional use or when the body has colds or infections.

Banana - Sweet flavour. It can create damp, phlegm and cold. Take these only when feeling hot and dry.

Melon - Sweet and mildly bitter flavour. It gently cleanses.

Mango - Sweet tasting. It builds fluid and cools. Avoid them if you are cold and damp or have phlegm in your nose or lungs. It is good for thirst and dry cough.

Pears - Mildly Sweet Flavour. It builds fluid and moistens.

Orange - Sweet and bitter tasting. It can cleanse and create dampness at the same time. Avoid if there is phlegm in your lungs or in your head. They are quite good for treating constipation.

Apples - Sweet and sour taste. They astringe, build fluid, tighten and tone the body.

Raisins, Dates and figs - Sweet tasting. They are over ripened fruits. They tend to nourish energy and blood.

Research by a team at the Horticulture And Food Research Institute Of New Zealand and published in the Journal Of Science Food And Agriculture, found that blackcurrants and boysenberries when tested on cultured human brain cells, blocked the cell damage that could lead to Alzheimer's disease.

A study published in the Journal of Agriculture And Food Chemistry reported that U.S. scientists who had fattened up hamsters on a high cholesterol diet and then fed them compounds of citrus peel from tangerines and oranges, saw a significant drop of 40 percent in their bad cholesterol levels.

A report by a team of scientists working for the U.S. Departments Of Agriculture found that in rodents, blueberries acted as effectively as a commercial drug lowering bad cholesterol.

Research appearing in the American Journal Of Medicine compared those who drank fruit and vegetable juice three times a week, to those who drank it less than once a week. They found that those who drank it more often, had a 76 percent decrease in rates of Alzheimer's compared to the group who drank it less.

Ohio State University researchers found that mice with blood vessel tumours, when fed a blueberry extract safely decreased the size of their tumours and improved survival rates. As reported in the Journal Anti-oxidants and Redox Signalling.

Researchers at Ohio University also found that black raspberries inhibit the development of oral, oesophageal and colon cancers in rats.

A research team from the Saint Louis University, found that breast cancer cells when treated with bitter melon extract significantly decreased growth and cell division. As published in the journal Cancer Research.

A study by researchers at the University of Michigan and published in the Journal Of Gerontology - Biological Sciences, found that rats fed a diet of grapes had lower blood pressure and improved heart function even though being fed a diet high in salt.

Scientists at the University of Reading found that by introducing blueberries to a regular diet, it resulted in improvements in memory, which may be beneficial to people with Alzheimer's disease. As reported in the Free Radical Biology And Medicine Journal.

Studies at the Ramban Medical Centre in Israel, showed that drinking a glass of pomegranate Juice daily, reduced the risk of cardiovascular disease. It slowed down cholesterol oxidation by almost half and reduced the retention of bad cholesterol.

A study by researchers at the University of California, published in the Journal Clinical Cancer Research, showed that drinking a quarter litre of pomegranate juice daily significantly slowed the progress of prostate cancer. PSA levels which indicate the rate the cancer is increasing went from an average of doubling every 15 months to doubling every 54 months in those who drank the pomegranate juice daily. This slowed the rate the cancer was growing by an average of over three and a half times.

A study by a team at the University of Kentucky, found that 76 percent of leukaemia cells were killed within 24 hours of exposure to a compound in grape seed in lab experiments. As reported in Clinical Cancer Research.

You will notice from many of the studies, how the bitter taste effectively purges unnatural and alien substances from the body, be they fats, toxins, phlegm or mutated cells.

Carbohydrates.

We have already discussed rice, which you should eat often. The others you can have for variety in your diet. Avoid ones with too much fibre and ones that are overly processed, as they are difficult to break down.

Bread can clog you up and usually causes most problems. Pasta and healthy cereals like porridge oats are better. If you are having a sticky porridge add berries or fruit juice to it, to help it pass more smoothly through your digestive tract.

Potatoes are slightly cooling and damp forming. You need to have a strong digestion to break them down. Avoid them if you have cold or damp type systems. Or you can add a small amount of spice to them to help them digest. If you really like them you can also mix a small amount of them with a portion of rice.

Oils And Fats.

We have previously discussed these. So we will just recap that the good ones are beneficial to the body and help things move more smoothly through it. They come from plants such as olive, sesame, rapeseed, hemp and sunflower. They are usually cold pressed and extracted with minimal processing. They are also found naturally in nuts, seeds and fish.

The bad ones generally block you up and are to be found in processed man made oils like hydrogenated vegetable oil and trans fats. They also come from animal fats, like red meat and dairy products.

You can even use the good oils externally. You can rub olive oil directly into your skin if it is dry, or into stiff and achy joints and muscles to ease pains and aches in them.

Nuts And Seeds.

These are highly nutritious and great for your body and general health. They are particularly good for hormones and fertility. They can also be effective at slowing down aging and are used in the regeneration of cells. They are great at reducing cravings and at keeping your brain and mood boosted with lots of essential nutrients. Pumpkin seeds and walnuts are best for hormones. Flaxseed is also a good all rounder with a good balance of omega oils in it.

However if you are blocked up with bad fats, then rich oils from the nuts and seeds can intermingle with them causing problems. Also if you are very hot, then these rich oils may be overcooked and can then turn into more heat, phlegm and toxins. So in this case, it is best to detoxify and cool down first with bitter tastes, and then introduce the nuts and seeds into your diet.

Stimulants.

Coffee, alcohol, spices, dark chocolate and red or black tea all produce heat and energy. They are the equivalent of petrol being poured on to a fire. It will produce a strong blast of flames but will burn and use up the logs more quickly. In the body stimulants will burn up anything available to give energy. This initially gives your body, mind and spirit a boost. However, in essence they are giving you energy at the expense of using up your reserves. In small amounts, when combined with more cooling, moistening, nutritious foods like vegetables, they can be very useful. They can provide extra power to break down these foods. They will burn some of them up, but will also extract the maximum nutrients from them. So in small quantities, they will give benefit.

Alcohol can be made from many different sources. All of these will give the alcohol extra unique qualities along with its base of heat and activity. Wines made from grapes tend to have heating and bitter qualities. Coffee and dark teas are the same. If you have a clean, phlegm and toxin free body, then these will just heat and dry fluids. But if you do have a poor diet and have gathered phlegm and toxins within, then these will most likely bake and congeal them into smaller more dangerous elements. You will notice in the many Western studies on alcohol and coffee, that one study suggests they are good, and the next says they are bad. As you can now understand, it all depends on the type of people you put them into. Generally they are bad for people who are already hot and toxic. And good for those who are cold and deficient in energy.

Spices create heat and movement in general. And power up and clear mucus from the lungs. However, their unique flavours can also cause many different actions in the body. Ginger is good for the stomach. Garlic and turmeric are good for blood circulation and cinnamon is good for creating hormones.

There are many sauces created from spices. These are fine to use in moderation as long as chemicals haven't been added. Of course the same rules apply in regards to the heat of the sauce. The more intense it is, the more dramatic effects on the body. So always try to balance it in a meal, say with lots of cooling vegetables or against the larger patterns existing inside or outside of your body, that is levels of cold and heat that are present.

Green herbs tend to have many active properties but are generally more balanced than spices. Some even having cooling properties as well.

Peppermint.

Peppermint is wonderful for the digestion. It is easy to take as peppermint tea. But if you can't take that, then try temporarily taking peppermint sweets until you acquire a liking for its flavour.

It moves, cleans, warms and then cools. Just like when you eat a peppermint sweet, it causes an active sensation in your mouth. It can become fiery and then feels like a cool breeze. It helps to create energy in the stomach and intestines. It cleans them, then cools them and leaves them fresh and ready, prepared for the next meal. You can even use it to gargle and clean your mouth and freshen your breath. Just like you see it being used in many bottles of mouthwash. It is great for treating many digestive disorders, particularly those involving gas, bloating and pains. You should have a cup of it after every meal.

A study by scientists at McMaster University published in the British Medical Journal reported that 40 percent of sufferers of irritable bowel syndrome found their symptoms disappeared after taking peppermint oil. They also found that taking bran, rich in fibre, did not improve their symptoms.

Green Tea.

There have been hundreds of studies on Green Tea. All of them suggest that it has excellent properties for activating, cooling and cleaning. It generally has a mild bitter taste. But some green teas can be more intensely flavoured. If it is mild, you can take many cups of it a day. It will cleanse and strengthen the digestive system. And also filter through the rest of the body, gently cleaning it as well. It is recommended to have a small cup after each meal. You can mix both peppermint and green tea together, and drink them from the same cup.

Green and darker teas like red or black have all come from the same plant. The difference is that green is fermented less in the processing of the tea. This leaves much more vitamins and minerals in it, giving it cooler properties. These heavier cooler qualities have been burnt out of the darker teas, leaving only heating and stimulating properties behind.

Researchers in Rochester found two chemicals in green tea which inhibit activity linked to causing cancer.

University of South Florida researchers found a component of green tea when fed in large doses to mice with similar characteristic plaques as found in the brains of Alzheimer's patients, reduced these plaques by as much as 54 percent. As reported in the Journal of Neuroscience.

A study in the Journal of Cancer Prevention Research found that men who were fed Polyphenol E. The equivalent to be found in drinking 12 cups of green tea per day, reduced their P.S.A. levels, a marker for the growth of prostate cancer, by 30 percent after 34 days.

Researchers from the University Of California concluded in a report, published in the International Journal Of Cancer, that women who drank more than 3 oz. of green tea per day had a 47 percent reduced risk of breast cancer, in comparison to those who drank no green tea.

A study from the UCLA School of Public Health and the Johnson Comprehensive Cancer Centre found that consumption of green tea reduced the risk of stomach cancer by 48 percent.

A report appearing in the Annals of Epidemiology found a statically significant reduction in the levels of bad cholesterol from the consumption of green tea, in a study of 13,916 participants.

Beans, Legumes And Pulses.

There are many different types. Such as aduki, soy, butter, mung, black, broad and kidney beans. And also chick peas, red and green lentils and so on. They are great foods filled with proteins, minerals and amino acids. They can be used as building blocks in the maintenance and regeneration of cells in the body. Many beans have as much or nearly equivalent levels of proteins in them as meats do. Soy beans have the highest level of protein.

You must however, pay extra attention to really chewing beans into a fine paste in your mouth, as they are quite hard to digest. You can also throw a little stimulant like spice in with them to aid your digestive system in breaking them down. Split lentils are a particular favourite as they are easy to cook and very high in protein. When mixed in with rice they will form a complete protein. The meal will contain all the essential amino acids the body requires. You can also put them with rice and spices into tasty soups, to make a very nourishing meal.

Sweets.

Sweet tasting foods like honey, liquorice and raw cane sugar can provide energy for the entire body. They will also hold food longer in the digestive tract, allowing it extra time to be broken down and absorbed. For this reason, liquorice is usually found in most Chinese Herbal Medicine formulas, to give the herbs more of a chance to be absorbed by the intestines.

Mildly sweet foods are particularly good for cold and energy deficient people. They will build them up and nourish their organs and mind. However if people have toxins and phlegm in them, then sweet and sticky food will bind the toxins into the body and even help to create more of them. So sweet food should be used appropriately to balance the body and in moderation.

Obviously, reduce levels of processed sweets and refined sugars. Sugars that have been heated into toffees and very sticky sweets will cause the most problems in the body. Try to avoid these. Eventually when you are eating healthily and balancing nutrients and energy. You will find it very easy to give up junk foods. In fact, you will find it becomes a natural progression, and very little effort, if any is required to break any dependant link on them.

Animal Products.

Let's start with red meat. From a Chinese Medicine perspective it is seen as a rich food naturally high in fatty oils, which gives it warming and phlegm creating properties. Both beef and lamb fall into this category.

As we have discussed, the Chinese and many other Asians, historically, have eaten animal products in small quantities. From none at all, up to one or two pieces a week. More affluent Chinese in some cities, ate more meat and richer foods. But physicians noted, as they ate these higher intakes, that their incidences of illnesses increased as well. So Chinese advice is to limit intake of meats in general to keep you healthier. Everything you can get from meat, you will often find in a much more easy to digest form, elsewhere in nature. Such as nutrients from vegetables and proteins from beans.

Many modern studies now confirm that less meat is better for us. In fact the more meat we eat, the more likely you are to shorten your life, suffer from cancer, heart disease and many other ailments.

A United States Federal study of over half a million Americans, between the ages of 50 and 71 years old, found that those eating the largest amounts of meats suffered from more heart disease and cancer, compared to those eating the least daily. Men had a 22 percent higher risk of dying from cancer and a 27 percent higher risk of dying from heart disease. In women, it was 20 percent higher from dying of cancer and 50 percent higher from dying of heart disease.

Findings in the American Journal of Epidemiology have shown that people eating more than 10 portions of red meat per week have nearly 50 percent higher chance of deterioration of the retina in old age, which can lead to blindness.

A University of Leeds team found that women who ate 57 grams of red meat daily had a 56 percent higher risk of breast cancer, compared to women who ate none. As reported in the British Journal of Cancer.

A study in the Journal of the National Cancer Institute by the National Institutes of health, of over a half million people, concluded that men who ate the most fat from red meat and dairy products had 53 percent increased risk of pancreatic cancer and women had 23 percent increased risk.

Next up we have fish. Fish used to be a very clean, non fattening healthy food. It contains good quantities of our friendly helpful omega oils. Unfortunately, factories have polluted our air with chemicals and vapours of mercury. Mercury is highly poisonous. It cools over cold seas and falls back to the earth. It is then absorbed by algae in the ocean. The fish eat the algae and we eat the fish. If we eat too much we can end up with high levels of dangerous mercury in us. Because of this, government agencies now recommend we limit our fish intake to two or four pieces per week.

We will discuss the problems surrounding mercury in more detail later on in the book.

When you are buying fish for omega oils, make sure you get wild fish. Wild fish get their oil form eating natural algae. Farmed fish are fed differently and have far fewer essential oils. They can be raised in underwater cages, containing up to 50,000 fish in each. Often they end up eating and breathing from the same water which is contaminated with their own wastes. Because of this, they are constantly fed antibiotics, hormones and other drugs.

Chicken and turkey are considered lean meats and are neutral in temperature. They are viewed as nourishing and strengthening. In China, organs and all other parts of the animals are used. Nothing is wasted. Often the Chinese will make a soup out of chicken bones to release all the extra nutrients from the marrow of the bones. They will use soups like these to strengthen individuals during and after illnesses. Once you have trimmed the fat, pork is also considered to be lean, healthy and nourishing.

Eggs are to be considered very nourishing and are said to support the Jing essence and the hormones in the body. They build energy, blood and nutrients. In the West, per gram, they are seen as one of the most nutritious foods you can eat. If you cut back on other animal products, then you should increase levels of eggs. If you have given up meat for moral reasons, then it is still ok to eat organic eggs. They have not been fertilized and will therefore not hatch into living chicks.

Wild game animals are always seen as far healthier than farmed ones. They are free to roam and eat a variety of different natural foods. Because they naturally move more the meat contains far less fat. Another aspect is that many farmed industry raised animals are often raised in inhumane conditions, leading to stress and disease, so they are often fed food containing antibiotics and hormones.

Before We Leave This Chapter.

It is interesting to note, that the foods that are sticky and slimy, like sugars, fats, greases and dairy, seem to have the effect of blocking up the circulation in our bodies. This interferes with the movement of nutrients and oxygen to cells and the extraction of waste from them. It also overburdens and puts pressure on organs, causing them to weaken, tire out and even rupture and scar. This in turn leads to most of our modern Western illnesses. Whether it is fats blocking our arteries and causing heart disease, or fats and toxins blocking our minds causing dementia, or toxins blocking and rotting our cells causing tumours and cancer.

Whereas, the big defenders against this stickiness, toxins and phlegm are our bitter tasting fruits and green tea, which purge away this garbage from our systems, and allow everything to move more freely again.

When we have rid ourselves of toxins and phlegm, we can start to reduce our intake of bitter tastes. And by increasing neutral flavours, we can fill our bodies up with all the necessary building blocks for their constant cellular regeneration. This will slow down ageing. And also feed, fortify and strengthen our minds and emotions.

Chapter Twenty Nine - General Foods And Tips For Your Daily Diet.

Start to look at your food differently, start to see it as a way of altering states in your body. Really taste your foods and assess their reactions inside of you. Are they heating you or are they cooling you. Are they detoxifying or moistening. Are they nourishing you, and so forth.

It will take time to develop sensitivity to their actions, but if you are persistent, this ability to see what they are doing will definitely come to you. And provide you with a great tool and lots of control to bring your body into balance and create good health.

When we have balanced bodies and are not using our foods medicinally to alter patterns such as heat or cold, then there are several foods we should always have in our diet. And several ways of eating we should always follow.

The Things We Should Do Are ...

Have a big breakfast, medium sized lunch and small sized dinner.

Try to eat in a consistent way, avoiding large gaps where your energy levels are being allowed to fall without being refuelled. If this happens you are more likely to want the wrong types of foods, such as high energy sugars and fats. These will only end up leaving a mess in your body and eventually making you sick. Try to keep your energy levels reasonably high on good quality clean foods.

Eat more slowly and chew your food into a paste. This will save you and your digestive system a lot of energy.

If we can save a little energy here and there by doing things in a smarter way, we will find that all these little savings start to mount up and we are now living with a reserve of energy. Remember energy is vital for everything in the body. It feeds and powers up all processes. Your heart, your brain and every other part of you is dependent on it. The more good energy you have, the better you will feel. Whether it is power for moving, talking, listening, thinking or staying in a positive mood. The more you have the happier and healthier you will be.

Avoid eating at night. However, it is fine to drink green tea or have fruit or fruit juice.

Avoid eating or drinking anything physically cold.

Avoid over eating. Try small more nutritious meals with nuts, seeds, eggs and so on. Rather than eating large meals which leave no room for digestion to work properly.

Try to have a varied diet, with at least a little taste of each flavour.
Avoid intense flavours.

Avoid eating dairy products, milk, cheese, yoghurts, cream and butter. Particularly those that come from cows.

In Your Daily Diet, Try To Include ...

Some bitter tasting fruit or juice. The more medium flavours like pomegranates, grapes and berries are the best and most productive in our systems. Generally, the more toxic we are the more we should have. The more clean we are, the less we need, as they are now flushing good nutrients away.

Have small amounts of highly nutritious foods like nuts, seeds, eggs and good oils. These will nourish, feed, help rebuild and lubricate our bodies. A simple way to see if you are running low on good oils, is to check for symptoms like dry skin, brittle nails and creaky joints making clicking sounds. If you have these you need more lubricating oils.

Have at least one portion of white rice a day. Preferably with vegetables. If your energy is low, have two portions. Add to it small amounts of spices like garlic, ginger, mustard or turmeric to enhance your digestion. You will need more of these in a cold winter and less in a hot summer.

We should have a mix of green tea with peppermint after meals and throughout the day. This will cool, clean and freshen our digestive tracts and also filter and cleanse the rest of our bodies.

The above are simple little tips that you can incorporate quite easily into your daily routine. You can start slowly and over time add each and every one of them in. By doing this, you will feel better right now and in the future, you will avoid many of the deadly illnesses which now plague our modern society.

Section Four - Breathing.

Chapter Thirty - The Breath Of Life.

"For breath is life, and if you breathe well you will live long on the earth" - Sanskrit proverb.

The very first thing we do when we enter this world, is open our mouths and pull in air. Simply, without it we die. While we are here, the better we can breathe, the more life we will fill ourselves with. When we breathe poorly, our minds and bodies suffer, we become tired and sluggish, even sleepy. When we are revitalised with air, we become alive, awake, alert, even brimming with life.

Air and its components, such as oxygen, are energetic and explosive. We only have to look in nature at the affects of air on fire to see its power. If we blow on hot embers and coals, we can make them glow with energy. Another example is a bellows, which can be used to strongly increase and fan the flames into a more raging fire.

To the Chinese, the symbol for Qi energy, is made up of two parts. One we have already learnt is food, particularly rice, and the other is air. Food and air are the essentials for life. Air invigorates, it brings things to life. It feeds the body, the mind and even the spirit.

The Chinese have developed a whole art form called Qi Gong. It is so important that it will have a whole section dedicated to it later in the book. For now all we need to know is that it is used for the cultivation of energy. Proper breathing is absolutely fundamental to its successful practice.

The Chinese are not alone in their respect for the benefits of maximizing breath. The Indians too, have developed their own techniques to gather energy and power through breathing. The Indian name for energy is Prana. Practitioners of Yoga and meditation use techniques to cultivate and refine energy through the breathing methods of Pranayama.

In the West, we have no such techniques, we simply ignore and are unaware of the massive benefits we can achieve from making proper breathing a part of our lives. The closest we get to deep breathing is through exercise. But this has its drawbacks and can also reinforce poor and unnatural breathing habits.

The impact of the proper breathing method described at the end of this segment has far and wide reaching implications right through the entire body and mind. When performed correctly, it will boost your energy levels, giving every organ and cell inside of you more life force, power and therefore more ability to carry out their duties with ease. Your mind will function with more clarity and your mood will be lifted and become less affected by external influences. When you flush your bloodstream with oxygen and energy you may even find feelings of happiness and a mini high. This is often experienced by Qi Gong, Yoga and meditation practitioners.

Because of its multiple benefits, it would be crazy not to incorporate, this natural breathing technique into your life. It will only cost you a little of your time, effort and patience. But will pay you back with so much good health in return.

Chapter Thirty One - The Components Of Air.

Air.

Our air is composed of approximately 21 percent oxygen, 78 percent nitrogen and about one percent other gasses. When we exhale, we breathe out about 5 percent less oxygen than we took in. This has been replaced with carbon dioxide and other waste materials from inside of our bodies. The 21 percent oxygen levels can vary depending on your environment. In cities with more noxious gasses there can be considerably lower levels.

Because our modern world has polluted the atmosphere. Destroyed our rainforests and other green areas producing oxygen. Our levels of it have actually reduced over the last hundred or more years. This means, that it has become even more vital to take every opportunity through proper breathing, to maximize our extraction of oxygen from the air into our systems.

Ions.

In Western terms, one of the vital components of the air, is electrically charged particles called negative ions. These are created wherever energy is transferred into the air. They are generated by waterfalls, thunder and lightning, the movement between wind and rain and so forth. The suns' ultraviolet rays creates them in abundance in the ionosphere, a band of ions gathered between 60 and 100 kilometres above the earth.

Negative ions are basically spare electrical charges. They help us in a number of ways. They attach themselves to and neutralize positively charged pollutants in the air such as chemicals, smoke, dust and toxins. This causes them to be dragged from the air to the ground, thus cleaning it. The other affects they have is the reaction inside of us. In the West they would say, they help to accelerate the delivery of oxygen to our cells, tissues, organs and brain. In the East they would say they charge and strengthen our Qi energy.

In unpolluted natural environments like mountains and the countryside, there are massive amounts of negative ions to be found. Mountainous air has about 5,000 ions per cc. The countryside has about 2,000 ions per cc. But as pollution rises in cities, it generates more positive charges, consuming the good negative ions. Dropping their levels to about a mere 50 ions per cc. In the East to combat this, office blocks widely use ionisers to increase levels of the good ones to more healthy amounts.

To feel the impact of positive ions on the body, think of how groggy, oppressed and uncomfortable you can often feel just before a thunder storm. At this time there are unusually high saturations of positive ions. If you do live in the city and feel sluggish where you work or in your home, it would be wise to invest in a negative ioniser. This will help replenish your environment.

Chapter Thirty Two - The Lungs.

The lungs are like an internal extension of your skin. Inside them, they create a vast network of air passageways that resemble tree branches. These become smaller and smaller until they reach tiny alveoli air sacs, about 300 million of them, which transfer oxygen and carbon dioxide in and out of the lungs and blood vessels. The lungs contain a massive surface area, about 750 square foot. That's around 35 times the surface of the skin.

Our lungs perform two major vital functions in the body.

Firstly, they pull in air, pass it into our blood and help with the heart to pump it around the body. The air then helps to empower and create our Qi, which provides the life force energy for our systems.

Secondly, they are one of the main components of the bodies waste disposal system. Every time you exhale, you are getting rid of significant amounts of fluids, carbon dioxide and other toxins from the blood. The blood filters absolutely everywhere through your body, gathering toxins and waste from cells, and also holding any improper or undigested particles coming from the digestive organs.

When you breathe the lungs put oxygen into your blood and take away this waste. You can easily see the amount being removed from your lungs by breathing on a mirror or a piece of glass. You can quickly see the moisture condense and build up on it. At the same time with this moisture, gas particles are also being emitted into the air. You take around 15 to 20 thousand breaths every day. Now if you start to multiply that by what you see on the mirror after only a few breaths, you can see the huge amount of waste that is being cleared from your body through your lungs. If you are not breathing deeply the waste is not being removed but is instead starting to build up in your blood making it and you toxic.

Lung Disorders.

Obviously in order to be able to breathe fully, we need to have strong healthy lungs. There are many things that can weaken our lungs and cause problems in them. The most common pattern you see in the lungs is phlegm. Part of the functioning of the lungs is to expel phlegm and fluids out of it when we exhale. If the lungs are unsuccessful in doing this, the phlegm can start to gather in them and block up their openings, which are the throat, mouth, nose and sinus cavities.

Phlegm can come from a number of areas. Such as a weak digestive system which can allow heavier improperly digested particles into the blood stream. These are pulled into the lungs for expulsion, but instead get stuck there and start to congest them. The food that seems to create the most phlegm in the lungs is cows' dairy products, such as milk, cheese, cream, butter and yoghurts. I have seen many lung problems and sinus disorders resolve dramatically from the removal of this one type of food alone from the diet. If you do so, you will generally start to feel the effects of reduced phlegm after a week or two. But be patient, it can take up to three months for it to be removed from all the tiny sacs and branches of the lungs. Other common phlegm creators are bananas, orange juice and rich sticky foods.

To further reduce the production of phlegm you may also want to avoid any physically cold foods and drinks. Always have hot meals or hot drinks with cold foods such as salads and sandwiches. Also avoid over eating, so you leave enough space in your stomach to properly digest your food.

When the phlegm in our lungs is cold it will remain clear or white and usually there will be plenty of it. If it is heated it tends to thicken and rot, turning yellow, green or darker. This type of mucus is often more prone to infections, as it is warm and a rich feeding ground for bacteria. Coffee, alcohol, cigarettes and the over consumption of spices can all generate heat in the lungs. Stress, frustration and anger are also common activators of heat. They tighten the rib cage and restrict movement through the lungs causing energy inside of them to rev up and generate heat.

Other emotions can also have a detrimental effect on the lungs. Grief, sadness, heartache, loss, disappointment, regret can all weigh heavily on them. The first thing you notice when someone is depressed, is the sunken chest and stooped bent forward shoulders. With this posture, the lungs cannot possibly work effectively. They will be unable to fully exchange carbon dioxide and other toxins for good fresh energy providing air. Therefore in this poor posture they may be helping to prolong the person's depression.

In general these types of emotions prevent the uptake of energy in the body, so they tend to cool it. However, they can easily mix with internal heat from the diet or with other emotions like stress, and anger. This then creates a mixed hot and cold pattern in the body.

When there is a lack of oxygen in the blood and weakened or congested lungs are unable to rectify this, people suffering from lung disorders may often feel suffocated and threatened. This can sometimes lead to paranoid or defensive behaviour. This in turn can lead to further stress and more complications for the lungs. As is often seen elsewhere in the body, everything is interconnected, so once you weaken one area, it can have knock on effects on others, leading to a further downward spiral and vicious circle of illness.

Our modern world has also played a significant part in lung disorders. Apart from the phlegm and toxins to be found in the food we eat. And the fumes, unnatural gasses and pollution in the air we breathe. It has also changed the work and play environment for most people. We are spending more and more time inside, working at desks in our homes and offices. Playing computer games, watching television or using the internet. All of these practices deprive us of fresh air and gentle exercise. Often is the case, that they cause us to slouch or lean over desks or keyboards, cramping and squashing our lungs up, preventing them from opening and inhaling and exhaling properly. It is very easy to see the importance our lungs play in our well being from this type of action. We easily become tired and our brains seem to slow and falter. Our whole bodies seem to become sluggish. During this activity, if you take a break and go outside or stand by an open window and breathe deeply, you will find within a matter of a few short minutes, that you become fresh, alert and awake again. Once the oxygen and energy have been pushed back into your blood stream and circulated around your body everything livens back up.

Constipation can create a big problem for the lungs. As toxins and waste material aren't being cleared by the bowels, the lungs come under pressure to take up the slack. The lungs can be overwhelmed by the extra work load and can often become blocked up. A common side effect of the lungs becoming hot and toxic on the inside is skin disorders. Acne, psoriasis and dermatitis can all come from heat and toxins in the blood. The blood should moisten and feed the skin, but if it has become overheated, it dries, inflames and agitates the skin. If it is toxic, it can try to push these toxins out through the pores normally used for sweating and managing the bodies temperature. The toxins and phlegm often become lodged in the pores, damaging and infecting them. This often produces acne and wet rashes. Until the lungs are cleared and cooled and have dispersed the heat and toxins from them, the blood will not be able to cool itself and rid itself of the toxins it contains.

Smoking.

One of the most damaging things you can do to your lungs, and to the rest of you, is to smoke. Smoking puts large amounts of both heat and dangerous chemicals into your lungs. Your lungs then help to distribute this into your blood where it can pollute the rest of your body. Smoking is a stimulant and therefore burns up nutrients and other sources of fuel inside of you. It will age you, damage your skin and organs, make your mind race and most likely prematurely send you to your grave. The biggest threat comes from cancer. Smoking is responsible for almost 90 percent of all deaths from lung cancer. In the United Kingdom, less than 10 percent of all patients survive it for longer than 5 years. Lung cancer is the most common form of cancer in the world. More people die from it than any other form of cancer. However, smoking doesn't just cause it, smoking has also been linked to playing a part in most other types of cancer as well.

What smokers don't realize is that part of the feel good enjoyment of having a cigarette is simply coming from the deep inhalation of air. This sends oxygen up to your brain, stimulating it and calming it at the same time. When people are trying to give up cigarettes, they should eat high energy and nourishing foods like white rice, eggs, nuts and seeds. This will support their minds and bodies. They should also take in peppermint, spices and bitter juices to clean, expectorate and stimulate their lungs.

Another reason to quit smoking is Chronic Obstructive Pulmonary Disease. This type of lung disease incorporates lung illnesses such as emphysema and bronchitis. It is the sixth most common cause of death in England and Wales each year, killing more than 30,000 people annually.

A study appearing in the journal Thorax, followed smokers over a 25 year period. They all had initially healthy lungs at the beginning of the study, but from smoking 25 percent of them developed clinically significant Chronic Obstructive Pulmonary Disorder and a further 15 percent showed signs of the condition, over the life of the study.

Yet another reason to give up smoking has been provided by a study from the Minnesota University, appearing in the Journal Of Neurology, Neurosurgery And Psychiatry. It found that smokers aged between 46 and 70 were 70 percent more likely to suffer from Alzheimer's disease as they aged, than those who had never smoked.

If you give up smoking, after a year you will have lowered your risk of many cancers and other lung problems. For an average smoker, their risk of lung cancer after quitting, is expected to return to that of a non smoker after about 10 to 15 years. But this is dependant on the amount and length of time that they have smoked. If they have smoked excessively for a long time then they may be left with elevated risks. However, by giving up they are still having a very positive impact on their lungs and are lowering that risk and increasing their overall health.

Proper breathing and some of the other techniques we are about to discuss, will help alleviate and reduce many lung disorders. Including other conditions such as asthma, emphysema, bronchitis, sinus and nasal congestion, and even excessive sneezing and yawning. The mind too will receive a boost from the extra oxygen and energy it gets, helping to relieve depression and low moods.

The immune system is very closely linked to the lungs in Chinese Medicine. Allergies, hay fever, colds and flu can all come about from a weak immune system. The link is quite straight forward, when the lungs are weak and have not created sufficient energy in the body, then the immune system too has not enough energy and is incapable of taking the immediate action of powering up production of white cells when the body is under some form of attack by a bug, bacteria or virus. The body is left undefended and the bug takes a hold in it.

Allergies and hay fever are often complicated by both a weakened immune system and phlegm in the lungs. When pollen, fumes or some other allergen starts to be inhaled, they quickly block up and overwhelm the already congested lungs and the rest of the system which can lead to inflammation and other problems.

Chapter Thirty Three - Abdominal And Complete Breathing.

In the West, people have developed a very unnatural way of breathing. This has come from several different reasons.

Firstly, we have poor posture. People are now often sitting hunched at desks while working, studying or using the internet and computers.

The old Western habit of bottling up emotions has also led to the lungs becoming tight, and stifling the energy as it moves through them. As young children when we had a problem we roared crying, throwing our arms in the air and letting everything go. Then we quickly got over it and became happy again. However as we aged we were criticized, ridiculed and made fun of for crying and expressing our emotions. So rather than letting them be over and done with. We started to hold them inside. Storing them up, where they would cause pain, obstruction and future illness.

This rigidity from incorrect upbringing stays with some people as they travel through their lives. It is very easy to spot a stressed person. One of the first things you will notice about them, is that they are holding themselves tensely and barely breathing. Apart from the long term damage that this is doing, in the short term, their brain won't be able to receive enough oxygen, which will stop it from thinking clearly and further escalate their problems.

Finally, another damaging habit we have developed, is the fashionable obsession of having a big chest and a tiny waist. This has led many men and women to pull and hold in their abdomens while puffing out their chests. This is probably the biggest cause of poor breathing habits in the West.

Unfortunately, as we age, this inadequate breathing pattern tends to worsen, our breathing becomes more and more shallow. Eventually breathing through just the top two lobes of the lungs. These can hardly supply the needy oxygen and energy demands of the body. Which will inevitably, if not corrected, not just reduce our standard of living and happiness, but also hasten our demise.

So what way should we breathe ? Well, the proper way, complete breathing, is to expand both the belly and the lungs as you take each breath in. Then let the lungs deflate back into place and at the same time, pull the belly in to its original starting position. If you look at animals, children or babies asleep, you will quite often see their abdomen naturally move up and down in a similar fashion as they are breathing.

The benefits of complete breathing.

It increases the amount of oxygen and energy being delivered to your blood. By breathing correctly, you can add extra litres of air with every inhalation. This enhances and refreshes every single part of you. Your organs, tissues and muscles will have more power and ability to do their jobs. Your mind, which requires the most oxygen, will feel more awake, alert and calm. This allows you more control of your emotions. You can be in charge of them, rather than them leading you. Your concentration, memory and thought processing will all become more sharp and heightened. Also by keeping your sinus cavities open and clear, it can help to circulate air beneath the brain, which can help to keep it and your emotions cool, particularly when it is overheating from the heat inducing emotions of anxiety, frustration and anger.

Your immune system will have access to a full reserve of energy. And when the body is threatened by bugs, it will easily be able to make all the white cells it requires. Thus successfully defending you against any bacteria, colds and flu.

Your energy levels will be increased, giving you more general get up and go. As your lungs have more capacity and can breathe more easily, you will be fitter and be able to do more. Your levels of stamina will excel.

As you require less energy from food, this will help you lose and manage your body weight more effectively. The actual massaging effect involved in correct breathing also massages the abdomen. Helping to push food down through the digestive organs and also drawing energy into them. This is again good for weight loss.

This action also massages the kidneys, and more importantly the adrenal glands. These are the most important producers of hormones in the body. This can stimulate them, clean them and help them make more hormones to heal, regenerate and power up all parts of you. The kidneys are of particular importance to the lungs. One of the hormones produced in the glands that sit on top of them is cortisone. Anyone who has asthma is aware of the importance of this substance. As most of the inhalers they sometimes depend on during asthma attacks, contain the very same stuff. In Chinese Medicine, when a practitioner treats asthma, they will treat the lungs, but will also strengthen the kidneys and therefore the natural production of cortisone.

This type of breathing also benefits the heart. Firstly it oxygenates the heart muscle. Then it packs blood with lots of oxygen thus reducing the amount the heart needs to get to cells, so the heart doesn't have to work as hard. And finally through this breathing, the lungs act like a bellows forcefully pushing blood through them and around the body. Again easing the workload of the heart.

Lastly the other big effect from complete breathing is the full exhalation. Oxygen and energy are exchanged for carbon dioxide, toxins and phlegm in the alveoli. By breathing deeply you significantly increase the size of this exchange. This will increase the amount of waste leaving your body. It will clean your blood and all parts of you. Leading to a much healthier and thriving system.

How To Breathe Properly.

The first step is to breathe through your nose for everyday normal breathing. This heats and moistens the air. So it is particularly useful in winter. However, if you find you are over heating, it is best to temporarily breathe through your mouth to cool yourself down and regulate your temperature. The tiny hairs in the nose also help to trap and filter, dust, toxins and other airborne pollutants. The sneezing mechanism is employed to eject bacteria and any other germs and invaders.

Up next is abdominal breathing. Between your lungs and the lower back is the diaphragm. This piece of tissue can be stretched to increase the capacity and volume of air into your lungs. To do this you will need to swell out your belly as you breathe in. This sucks the diaphragm down, massaging your lower organs and allowing more air into you.

When you breathe out, pull the belly in. This will push the diaphragm back up into your lungs, helping them to squeeze out any waste and fluids.

Until you get good at this, it is sometimes useful to practice by standing with your back against a wall. Then place your hand on your abdomen and feel it move out as you inhale and pull in tightly as you exhale. Over time you will find it easy to extend your belly in and out, moving it over four inches and more, every time you breathe.

Finally, when you are breathing through your nose and your abdomen is moving properly as well, you can then apply the last stage, which is to expand your chest as you breathe in and simply let it drop back into its lower position as you breathe out. Now in every breath you are completely maximizing oxygen and energy intake, and expelling waste as effectively as possibly from the lungs.

You will need to practice this daily for at least two minutes. It will eventually sink into your subconscious and you will find that it adopts it as your normal everyday method of breathing. In some people this will gradually happen over a month or two, some others however may take up to a year to perfect and retain this method. But no matter how long it takes, stick with it. Because of all the great benefits it will produce, it is definitely worth the small amount of practice that is required.

Chapter Thirty Four - Posture, Massage And Diet.

For the proper functioning and good health of the lungs, it is very important to maintain a fully open and erect straight posture. When you are stooped over reading, writing, using a keyboard and so on, you will end up squeezing down on your lungs and heart. This diminishes breath and blood circulation to your mind and body. The spine too can be affected, as nerves leading from it can be squashed. This can interfere with messages from the brain to organs and other parts of the body. Over time this crooked posture can begin to take hold and even when standing up, you may find that your spine and shoulders can be hunched over. Stress can also be a player here. Tensing and tightening your ribcage, pulling your lungs and spine out of its proper alignment.

Poor posture can have a very negative effect in your subconscious mind. Your subconscious has been formed from being fed repeated patterns of behaviour. It associates feeling down with stooped shoulders and lowered head. It associates frustration with tight and seized muscles. So when your head and shoulders are drooped, apart from the physical implications of not getting enough oxygen into your blood, your subconscious mind will also start to set up other negative actions, feelings and thoughts to play along with this weak posture. And you will find your mood becoming lower and lower.

Alternately if you are feeling down, if you stand upright and open your lungs and breathe deeply, you will find your mood starting to lift. This even works for something as simple as a smile. When you start to smile, the subconscious links this action with happiness and starts to generate a more positive state of being. It is simply following your physical actions. In another scenario, if you are physically tense your mind will become wound up. If you relax your muscles and body, calmness will start to return to your mind.

In this way, by consciously keeping good posture and smiling as often as we can, we will keep our body and mind at a higher level of health and happiness. A good way to develop and practice posture and smiling is through Qi Gong. If you don't practice Qi Gong, then just become as mentally aware as you can to the problem of poor posture. And every time you catch yourself slouching, stooping over, tightening up and even frowning, then correct yourself. Over time, with conscious effort and repeated practice, your subconscious will be imprinted with this better posture and will automatically assume it as the normal method of behaviour.

Massage.

A simple back massage is quite useful for strengthening and relaxing the lungs. By gently kneading the tissues, it brings extra blood flow, oxygen, energy, hormones and nutrients directly into them. Which over a period of time will help to build them up, increasing their power to function properly. Massage also loosens the tissues and muscles helping to reduce any damage from tension and stress. This can allow muscles to relax back into their correct positions and will aid good posture.

You don't have to be an expert to massage. Many simple techniques work as effectively as more complex ones. However, you should always be gentle and not hurt your patient. Being particularly careful not to press on the spine or the sides of it. The more gentle massages you get or give, the better. It is particularly useful for children with asthma. A daily back massage can have dramatic effects in reducing asthma occurrence in children.

Diet.

The spicy taste in small amounts can be very beneficial to the lungs. It can warm them and provide them with energy and power to function. But more importantly it helps them to expectorate fluids. This unblocks them and helps them operate more successfully. Once open, they can easily take in air, exchange it with toxic gasses and then push them out of the body. Spices will also keep the nose, sinus, throat and mouth open and phlegm free.

Spices in moderation can also help the digestive system. They can give it power and heat and dry up any phlegm in the intestines, preventing it from entering the lungs and the rest of the body.

However, big amounts of spice can overwork the lungs and wear their energy out. So use them in moderation.

The sour taste, such as apples and vinegar, can astringe, causing fluid to build up in the lungs. This is useful for dry conditions, such as dry cough and dry type asthma. But it is obviously unhelpful if you already have too much fluid or mucus in the lungs, nose or head.

The salty taste too, will astringe and moisten the lungs. Mangoes which are sweet and cold can produce fluid in the lungs. And orange juice which is sweet, bitter and cold, also has this effect. If the sweet taste is excessive, like lots of sugar, then the lungs can get sticky and blocked up.

Our final taste, is bitter, such as pomegranate, fruit or juice. It is useful for cleansing heat, phlegm and toxins from the lungs and the blood which filters through it.

Chapter Thirty Five - The Lungs, Things To Do And Things To Avoid.

To recap and summarize what we should and should not do for our lungs, we will break it down into the two categories below.

Things To Avoid.

Smoking. There is no surer general way to damage your lungs and increase your chances of dying from cancer or lung failure than from smoking. It will also prematurely age your skin and body. The best thing to do is give them up. It is obviously hard to quit smoking but it is one of the most important things you can do for your health. If you cannot, then drink lots of bitter juices. In particular green tea and pomegranate juice, but also berries and grapes and so forth. These will help to remove some of the heat and chemicals from the cigarettes in your blood and also in the lungs themselves.

Reading, studying, slouching, bending over at a desk and general poor posture. These will physically stifle your lungs, preventing them from inhaling air and exhaling toxins effectively. In this case, it might be difficult to give up your job or stop studying for an exam etc. So all you can do is become very mentally aware to try to always maintain good posture, where your lungs are unrestricted and can breathe freely. Also take as many breaks as you can and take deep breaths and stretch your lungs open during them.

Give up dairy. If you have phlegm on your lungs then cutting out dairy from your diet will dramatically reduce its quantity for most people. Replace milk with rice or soya milk. Replace butter with unprocessed extra virgin olive oil or other good plant oils. You can mix these oils with green herbs like basil and oregano for extra flavour if you wish.

Avoid and resolve constipation. If your bowels are blocked your blood will pull more waste and toxins into it. This can easily lead to your lungs becoming congested as they have to deal with the extra burden of waste to be disposed of.

If your lungs or sinus have too much mucus then avoid phlegm creating foods like bananas, oranges, mango and rich and sticky foods. Also avoid foods that retain fluids like apple, apple juice, vinegar and salt.

Add foods like white rice and mild amounts of spices into your diet to reduce and dry phlegm. Bitter juice like pomegranate and berries can also help to expel mucus and dry out your lungs.

Learn to control and manage your emotions. Details of how to do this will be given later. Emotions like grief, disappointment, heartache and even unfulfilled dreams and ambitions can all weigh heavily on the lungs and heart. This can cause your shoulders to droop and chest to collapse, which will stifle and damage your lung and heart energies.

Stress can also impact the lungs and weaken its energy. When you get stressed, you hold yourself tightly and the lungs will be unable to expand and deflate properly. Some people may find that they are holding their breath and barely breathing during times of stress. From this the ribs can even develop pains and aches, as energies and physical substances become caught and trapped in this area.

Things To Do.

Get yourself an ioniser. The more negative ions in the air around you, the more cleaner and pollutant free it will be. It will also electrically charge the air you consume, bringing this extra energy into your body.

Try to do more gentle exercise like walking out in the fresh air. This will stimulate the lungs and increase circulation through them. Qi Gong and Yoga are also excellent exercises for your lungs, body, mind and spirit.

Practice good posture and proper breathing daily, until it has become immersed in your subconscious. And has now become a natural habit and part of you.

Get a back massage as often as you can. This will bring energy, blood and hormones into the lungs boosting them up.

Chapter Thirty Six   -   The Common Cold.

Western Medicine sees colds very differently than Chinese Medicine does. They believe that colds are solely to do with exposure to bacteria and viruses.

Whereas Chinese Medicine believes that if a bug is really virulent, that many people may succumb to it and become infected. But in most cases for ordinary bugs that create common colds, the internal strength of the body, in particular the energy, is far more important to prevent them. If your energy is very strong you may even be able to avoid getting them altogether.

I can personally attest to this, as a practitioner of medicine I am constantly exposed to all types of germs yet rarely get an infection. Before I studied Chinese Medicine I used to get 3 to 4 colds a year. But since I began following its techniques and practising Qi Gong, I now hardly ever get any. And if I do it is always because I have failed to follow the theories correctly or that I was lazy and had skipped over my Qi Gong training for a period of time. So even from my own personal experience I know that catching colds is more about the strength of the energy inside of us than exposure to germs.

We are surrounded by bugs all the time. A study by a team at the University of Arizona, has shown that workers desktops have hundreds of times more bacteria on them than office toilet seats. They found desktops had 21,000 germs per square inch, compared to 49 germs per square inch of toilet seat. Office phones were even worse with 25,000 germs per square inch.

Another study by researchers at the University of Washington, found staph bacteria at nine out of ten public beaches it tested in the United States. Seven out of thirteen samples it tested were M.R.S.A.

And finally to further highlight the germs around us, a study by the London School of Hygiene and tropical Medicine took samples from 409 people at bus and train stations at five major cities in England and Wales. To their surprise they found that more than one in four people had bacteria from faeces present on their hands.

It is a fact that there are far more bugs present in our environment in summer than in winter. They breed far more easily in summer heat. They are just like flies and bigger bugs which you see swarming in hot and damp areas. And yet people generally get colds in winter, not in summer. So why does this happen ? It is, as the Chinese claim, simply to do with the strength of your bodies energy, rather than exposure to bugs.

In the cold weather, your body gets drained of its energy. There is not enough Qi to properly power up and run your immune system. The immune system always has some white cells active in the body searching for intruders. When the white cells find some, alerts are sent back to the immune system which then goes into a massive production of more white cells. It creates an entire army full of them, which are formed to hunt and kill the invaders. So in summer, because of the heat, you naturally have plenty of energy and this army is easily made. But in winter, if you have been standing out in the cold, the wind or the rain, then your energy levels have been drained. Cold will literally steal the life force from your body, and your immune system will have no power to make any army to defend the body. The bugs will simply then walk in and set up camp inside of you.

Researchers at the Common Cold Centre in Cardiff University, conducted an interesting experiment. They took 180 volunteers and got half of them to put their bare feet in icy water for a mere twenty minutes. They found that 29 percent of the people exposed to the icy water developed a common cold within five days, compared to only 9 percent of those who had not put their feet into the water.

Another study published in the Journal of Nutrition, by researchers at Michigan State University, found that mice when put on a calorie restricted diet found it harder to beat infections than those eating normal amounts. More of the under fed mice were infected, displayed more symptoms and took longer to recover, than the other properly fed ones. Their lack of food caused a reduction in energy, which caused their immune systems to fail to produce enough killer cells to fight off an infection.

Many of the symptoms of a cold are not actually caused by the bugs themselves, who simply want to feed off your body. But are created when your body tries to gather all its existing energy into your immune system, which leaves your circulation and other organs working very ineffectively. For example, when your digestive system loses its power. It will be unable to break down food properly. This leaves more waste and thicker particles behind. These get pulled through your blood, up into your lungs, where they start to congest them. Your weakened lungs don't manage to successfully breathe out these heavier particles, causing phlegm to build up in them and their openings, the sinus cavities and the nose.

The best thing to avoid colds is daily practice of Qi Gong. It brings your energy to such higher levels that most people who practice it, will be invulnerable to colds and infections. However, if you have not the time or patience to practice Qi Gong, then these other methods to keep your energy strong and protect you, are quite often successful.

Firstly, stay warm. When you are warm, you will have reasonable levels of energy in the body. When you get cold they get depleted. In winter, always wrap up warm. Wear extra clothes. Leggings, gloves, scarves and hats can all hold energy and heat in your body, vastly reducing your likelihood of colds.

Avoid anything that really depletes your energy in cold weather. This includes things like over working and Western style exercise.

Grief, disappointment and sadness can all have a detrimental effect on your lungs, collapsing them and drooping your shoulders. This reduces your ability to breathe and receive the energy you need from the air, leading to reduced power and ability in your immune system. Practice proper posture and the breathing techniques discussed previously to alleviate this.

Next up, avoid phlegm producing foods, which can block up your body, wasting the precious energy it needs to run the immune system. The phlegm itself can also create great breeding and feeding grounds to harbour bacteria in. If you give up dairy products, you will find a reduction in the number of colds you get each year. You will also find you get less mucus if you do get a cold. And it will not last as long as normal.

Any foods that create heat and energy are useful in preventing and dealing with colds. But don't overuse them. As this can lead to problems and illnesses from internal heat. Studies on alcohol, spices and hot herbs like Ginseng, have shown the participants taking them get colds less frequently than those in the studies who did not consume them.

Actions To Take If You Think You Are Getting A Cold.

If you do feel a cold coming on in winter, then get as much rest as possible. Avoid any strenuous activity which will drain away energy from the immune system. Keep yourself warm and avoid exposure to cold. Every few hours, take small amounts of hot drinks like coffee and alcohol to give your energy a boost. Spicy dishes can be helpful as well. They will provide energy and also help to expectorate and push the germs out of your body.

Avoid phlegm creating fluids like dairy and rich foods. Reduce cold creating foods like water and even bland vegetables and sweet fruits, until you feel well again. Any excess fluids will have the effect of piling up in your system and create more mucus.

Bitter fluids like pomegranate, bitter berries and grapefruit and lemon mixed with water, can be helpful with a cold. Although these juices are cooling in nature, they are also good at purging unwelcome guests from the body. These juices help to attack the bacteria, preventing it from getting a foot hold in your body and quickly forcing it out of you. Always heat these juices up or add hot water from the kettle to them. Otherwise the cold juice will steal energy from you.

However, if you do not have mainly cold symptoms but instead a hot fever, then it is important to balance the body by eliminating heating foods like coffee and alcohol. And also increase your intake of bitter, cleansing and cooling foods like cool or room temperature lemon and water or pomegranate juices.

M.R.S.A.

Multi-Drug Resistant Staphylococcus Aureus, as the name suggests is a bug that is very difficult to treat. It can often be very severe and even lead to death, being fatal in about 20 percent of people who develop m.r.s.a. blood stream infections and fatal in about 40 percent who develop m.r.s.a. pneumonia.

Surprisingly, it comes from Staph Aureus, which can be found in 30 percent of healthy people, causing them little or no problems at all. So why does it become so dangerous and life threatening in some people ? Because these people have weakened their energy in their bodies to extremely low levels. For example in hospitals, people may have undergone surgery, which has cut and sliced through their tissues and organs. Every part of their energy system is now trying to recover and rebuild this damaged area. Leaving no power available for their immune system. So a simple bug turns into a life threatening one. Strong antibiotics can also play a part in weakening patients. As although on the one hand it is trying to flush the bug out of a patient, on the other, it is also sometimes flushing away all their natural and immune energy too.

If you have to have an operation or a stay in a hospital, then try to follow these guidelines. Firstly do everything you can to strengthen your energy before attending the hospital. Avoid foods that are damp forming like dairy. And when you are there, eat plenty of clean energy rich foods like white rice. Keep yourself as warm as possible, without being uncomfortable. Ask for extra blankets if needed. And finally perform energy providing breathing exercises as often as possible.

Section Five - Cancer.

Chapter Thirty Seven - Cancer.

Cancer is the second leading cause of death in most developed nations throughout the world. In England, it is responsible for over a quarter of deaths from all categories of illnesses. About one in three people can expect to develop some form of cancer within their lifetime. In general, cancer is increasing at an alarming rate. For example, in the U.K. between 1995 and 2000, malignant melanoma rates increased by 24 percent, uterine cancer by 22 percent, breast cancer by 12 percent, prostate cancer by 25 percent and non-Hodgkin's lymphoma by 17 percent.

However lung cancer, the most common form of cancer is decreasing. This is not due to better treatment but simply to reductions in the number of people who smoke. As the rate of smoking declines, there is a proportionate decline in deaths from lung cancer. Western science estimates that about 80 percent of cancer is preventable by avoiding smoking and making changes to diet, exercise and weight control.

Most people are unaware that cells can mutate in the body thousands of times over a lifetime. Cancers can appear and if the body is working well, natural killer cells from the immune system can neutralize these cancerous cells before they become out of hand. Certain compounds from foods are also known to slow down and inhibit growth of cancerous cells. Whereas others, such as bad fats, are known to do the opposite, to promote and help the growth of these abnormal cells.

From the Chinese perspective of the bigger picture, it is easier to see the causes of cancer, than it is from a Western viewpoint of isolating and reducing to the smallest levels of the cells. Cancer may begin from a single abnormal cell that starts to multiply out of control. Then with other like cells, it enlarges and forms tumours which invade healthy tissues around them. This may eventually disrupt the vital work of organs in the body.

The Chinese, however are more interested in how these cells became damaged and started to mutate in the first place. And of course, more importantly, how to avoid this happening. They believe that a combination of four factors come together to cause cancer. They are heat, toxins, stress and weak energy. It is not always necessary to have all four. But in most cases they will be present.

1) Firstly, we have toxins. Any type of toxic phlegm in the body may contribute to damaging the cells surrounding it. Just as we see decay in nature rotting and destroying living cells around it. Like a bad apple, which rots the good one beside it as well. Precisely what is happening at the

cellular level is more a matter for Western science. Perhaps the toxic gluey phlegm has impeded nutrition and oxygen from getting into the cells leading to changes in their DNA programming.

However regardless of the actual mechanism, phlegm and toxins are clearly a leading player in the cause of cancer. Many large scale Western studies have concluded that both chemical toxins and natural substances like fat from dairy and animal products without doubt increases risks of cancer.

2) Heat is another cause. It quite simply burns up and damages cells. An intense burst of heat may cause severe damage and even destruction to cells, such as through sun burn or exposure to radiation. Most people are unaware that radiotherapy, used to treat cancer, can in some cases cause new cancers to form at some stage in the future. It usually takes many years for this to happen. Just like a sunburn as a child may not cause cancer for decades and decades.

We again see heat being involved through our diet. Alcohol, which as we now know is hot in nature, can in excess dramatically increase risks of cancer. Smoking, a huge cause of cancer, pours heat and toxins into the lungs. Even sugar, which causes heat, increases the risk.

A study at the University of Umea in Sweden, involving 64,500 women, found that the top 25 percent with the highest blood sugar levels, had a 26 percent increased risk of developing cancer, in comparison to the 25 percent with the lowest blood sugar readings.

Other studies involving minerals like calcium and selenium, which produce cold in Chinese Medicine, have shown the opposite, reductions in rates of cancer. This is also true for the many studies relating to vegetables, a great source of cooling minerals. These strongly point to lower levels in cancer as consumption of vegetables increase.

An interesting study at the Children's Hospital of Philadelphia, appearing in the American Journal of Epidemiology, also linked heat with cancer. This time in brain tumours. Their study examined the parents of 318 children with brain cancer and the parents of 318 healthy children for comparison. They found that men who had been exposed to some form of intense heat from saunas, hot tubs, electric blankets or the like, in the three months before conception, were much more likely to become the fathers of the children with the tumours. The studies findings concluded that heat damages the genetic material in the sperm, which then passed on genetic mutations to any of their offspring.

Another study by scientists at the University of Tehran, published in the British Medical Journal, found that drinking hot tea, 66C to 69C, produced twice the risk of oesophageal throat cancer, when compared with drinking lukewarm tea, 65C or less. And drinking very hot tea, 70C or more, produced an incredible eight fold increased risk.

3) Stress impedes the movement and circulation through the body. As you tighten up with stress, everything gets trapped and caught up. This helps to increase the three other causes relating to cancer. Firstly, it traps toxins. As the body seizes and clamps down on them, they get more caught and embedded into you. Secondly, this tightness causes your energy to push circulation more forcefully through it, which causes you to heat up. Think of how hot and red faced someone gets when they are uptight, frustrated and angry. And finally, long term, the stress can wear out and weaken your entire body. Leaving your immune system weak and unable to destroy mutating cells.

4) If your energy becomes weak, your body has less power to clean away toxins that might damage your cells. Your immune system is also dependant on good levels of energy to produce the necessary killer cells needed to deal with mutations. Weak energy is usually the reason why cancer tends to appear in older rather than younger people, who naturally have more energy.

Summary.

Cancer is generally caused by a combination of heat, toxins, stress and deficient energy. To prevent cancer we should limit our exposure to extreme heat, such as sunburn, coffee, alcohol and cigarettes.

We should avoid foods that create phlegm and toxins, such as man made chemicals, sugars, dairy and animal fats.

We should include foods that cool us down, such as mineral laden vegetables.

We should consume plenty of fruit and juices, particularly those tasting bitter, like pomegranates, grapes and berries. These help us to detoxify and flush heat, phlegm, chemicals and dead and damaged cells from the body.

We should also learn how to relax and avoid stress. And keep our energy levels as high as possible in our systems.

Qi Gong is an excellent method to keep the body healthy and help prevent cancer. In China, Qi Gong therapy and exercises can be prescribed as part of the treatment for tumours and cancers.

If you do find yourself with cancer, you should take up Qi Gong or Yoga. Do daily complete breathing exercises. Learn how to manage your stress. And do as many relaxing activities as possible. Also clean your diet up. Completely avoid all toxins and phlegm producing foods. Particularly sugars, dairy and red meats. Take plenty of bitter fruit and juices to detoxify. And lots of white rice to keep energy levels high. And vegetables to build up cooling elements in the body.

Section Six   -   The Climate And The Seasons.

Chapter Thirty Eight   -   The Climate.

Traditionally the climate played a substantial part on impacting upon peoples health. You could imagine how difficult it must have been for someone who lived one or two hundred years ago, to suffer from an illness like the flu in the middle of a harsh cold winter. Living in a cold, poorly heated house, it would have been very difficult to get the energy needed in the immune system to create white cells to fight off the flu or even a cold. Or you could imagine how hard it would have been to get rid of a lingering chesty phlegm filled cough, living in an old damp house in the countryside during a freezing and wet winter. Suddenly, little illnesses could turn into big life threatening ones. Particularly for the elderly, or for people with pre-existing conditions or weak constitutions. You could envision also working out on the land in the wind or the rain, or in cold stone floored factories at the turn of the century.

This exposure to the harsh elements and extremes of nature would have been responsible for many diseases and even deaths in times of the past. Such was their importance, that Chinese doctors often referred to extremes of weather as external evils. They characterized these into cold, damp, heat, fire, summer heat, dryness and wind.

Nowadays, we are not so vulnerable to the climate. We have radiators and central heating to keep us warm in the winter. And air conditioning to keep us cool in the summer. Because of this, many of us have become complacent and unaware of just how damaging the weather can be. Even if we are no longer exposed to the extremes, we can still be badly affected by it. In this section we will explore different climates and seasons. We will see both the positive and negative effects they can bring to our bodies and minds. And we will see, once again, how we can use diet and other methods to bring balance and harmony to our systems to avoid any ill consequences from exposure to elements such as too much cold, heat, dryness and dampness.

Chapter Thirty Nine   -   The Seasons.

The seasons work in a yearly cycle to create a balance in nature. If things remained too hot for too long, they would start to dry up, burn up and eventually die. If things stayed cold and inactive, everything would become lifeless and nothing new would grow. So hot summers full of life and energy, where physical things start to get used up and become depleted, turn to cooler autumns and colder winters, where physical things start to gather and rebuild their essences. Then they lie dormant and wait for spring for new growth and blossoming to begin the cycle all over again.

In much the same way, this also applies to the human being. If we stay too physical and hot for too long we burn ourselves out, using up our fluids, energy and hormones. If we get too cold and inactive, things slow down and stagnate in our bodies. We become tired and lifeless. Even our minds can lose their buzz and sparkle. Everything in us and in nature constantly ebbs and flows back and forth in a cycle of events.

Although, modern technology has caused us to become somewhat out of sync with nature and the seasons, they still play a big part in our lives. Forcing us to change our lifestyles, becoming more active in summer and slowing down in winter. This helps our bodies stay balanced, not burning up too much nor at the other end of the scale, gathering too much.

In this chapter we will discuss this cycle further through each individual season. We will see ways they can help us and ways they can hinder and harm us.

Winter.

The benefit of winter, is that it gives our bodies a chance to slow, rest and cool down. This conserves and restores fluids and essences that have been used up during the hot summer months. As everything slows, including electrons in atoms, physical things start to huddle together, and congeal and thicken.

If we are wise and follow nature. If we eat and do the right things, we will allow the building blocks that support and renew our organs and bodies to become somewhat replenished. If however, we are reckless in winter. If we step out of line with nature or eat too many heating foods, instead of having a storehouse of nutrients for the year ahead, we will face it from an already weakened and depleted position.

So what should we do in winter ? Well we don't have to do to much extra. We can start by following the other healthy tips in the book. And then add in a couple of extra ones, to do with the weather.

Lack of sun, and the cold and damp are the main problems we have to face in winter. The cold is obviously caused by the earth rotating its position away from the sun. The sun has then less of a chance to provide energy to your part of the world. With less energetic charges in the air, there is less heat and everything becomes colder. With less heat to dry, everything starts to become more damp. Dew forms on the grass in the mornings. And condensation appears on the windows. When it rains, the puddles lie on the ground and as there is no heat to dry them, they are not evaporated and end up slowly sinking into it. The ground can then become waterlogged with mucky puddles.

Too much cold and damp in the body tend to weaken and block up your energy and circulation. Fluids will congeal and thicken. They can block up and impede the workings of your joints, your organs and even your mind. You tend to get symptoms like feelings of heaviness, tiredness and being weighed down. Your head can feel cloudy, your thoughts muddled and even a little confused. Your nose might feel stuffy or runny. And your mouth sticky or filled with phlegm. Your lungs may be congested and produce mucus. The digestive system may slow and cool, leading to even more thick fluids in the body and perhaps even indigestion and odourless loose bowel movements. All these problems will further reduce your already weakened energy reserves.

Energy levels reduce considerably in winter time. This is for a number of reasons. Firstly, the sun gives us less heat and energy. The external cold itself, will drain and pull energy from our warm bodies into it. And finally the body has to now waste its own energy, trying to create heat to balance the external cold.

Because of this drop in energy, and therefore the weakening of your entire system, most illnesses will become worse in winter, (however some conditions involving heat may actually reduce in intensity).

Cold causes things to contract and tighten, so as it gets into muscles and joints, it can cause them to seize and become painful. As energy and movement slow, the physical gathers, swelling and reducing space, causing pressure on nerve endings and leading to pain.

The lungs on exposure to cold air, can constrict and tighten severely, leading to increased occurrence of asthma and lung disorders.

Cold can leave the immune system weak and the body defenceless, as there is not enough energy to create white cells.

The mind too can also suffer, as there is not enough power to keep it stimulated and running at peak levels. Many people therefore experience a dip in mood in January and February as their energy reserves are running low.

To protect ourselves from the negative effects of cold in winter, it is quite obvious that we need to wrap up warmly, to wear lots of layers of clothes. Forget about fashion, your health is way more important. Make sure you have lots on you. Wear trousers, long johns, thermal underwear, hats, scarves and gloves, whatever it takes to keep you warm. If you start to get cold, you are quite simply letting the life force energy drain out of you. At this stage you should be starting to understand how important your energy is to your entire well being, so protect it from the cold as much as you possibly can.

If you were exposed to extreme cold, you could get hypothermia and die. But any exposure at all is still depleting you. So wrap up and keep warm when you are outside and inside. Follow all those old sayings your granny used to tell you. Don't go to bed with wet hair or sleep in draughts. Change out of wet clothes and so forth.

Next up we can introduce more warming and active foods into our diets. These will balance the external cold. You can add small amounts of spices and alcohol. But still be careful, if you get carried away and use too much, you can actually create excessive internal heat. This may aggravate your system and lead to illnesses. Also by overheating your body, you will undo the natural replenishing effect that winter has on you. So use heating foods in moderation. Just enough to bring you back into balance and avoid damage from over cooling.

Spring.

Everything starts back up in Spring. Leaves appear back on the trees, flowers start to peep out of the ground and come back into bloom. Animals wake up and come out of hibernation.

However for the human being, although it is a welcome time, with the sun and its energy returning. And all that has been stored and gathered over winter now being put to good use to rejuvenate the body, it can also be a very changeable and therefore dangerous time. The body and mind can be tricked into believing that the warm weather has returned. Because of this we turn the heating down and change our heavier, warmer clothes for lighter ones. Only to have the weather sharply swing back to the cold a week later, leaving many of us caught short and exposed to the climate. This can obviously weaken us and quite often causes problems like common colds.

It is again easy to avoid. Just be aware of it and keep extra clothes on you or within easy reach if the weather turns bad. Such as in your car or at your desk at work.

Summer.

At the beginning of summer, everything is lustrous, alive and in full swing.
The rays of the sun have fed the earth, energizing it, bringing forth life in all its full glory.

Then towards the end of summer, the earth may start to become dried up. Unable to keep up with all the demands of the moving and active energy. Plants may become starved of nutrients and water, and begin to wither.

Or if there has been an abundance of rainfall, the heat and damp may combine. This humid weather can bring an infestation of bugs and bacteria. All the processes of decay will speed up. Living things will become swamped by the fluid and heat, leaving them to rot and putrefy, providing feeding material for the bugs.

In the body all that damp and heat can lead to prime conditions for food poisoning and stomach bugs. Or even just digestive and general problems relating to heat and toxins. Such as smelly urine, odorous and urgent bowel movements, inflamed painful swellings and skin eruptions, toenail infections, body and foot odours and bad breath. All that phlegm and heat may congest and disrupt the organs and mind too. Leading to many problems for them.

If you begin to suffer from damp and heat conditions and cannot see a doctor then food is the best way to treat them. Avoid fats, rich foods and sticky sugars. Avoid heat producing foods like coffee, spices and alcohol. Instead take in plenty of bitter fruit and juices like pomegranate, grapes and berries. Lots of green and peppermint tea too. These may make your bowel movements more odorous at first, as they use it as an exit to purge and clean your system. But stick with them and you will find yourself feeling much fresher and better after a while. You will find that your energy levels perk up too. As all that congested heat and damp wasn't just blocking you up but had also been draining your energy away, as your organs had to work much harder to push everything through them. The heavy feeling from the excess of damp fluids gathered in your body will also disappear, leaving you feeling lighter, with lots of get up and go.

Summer heat can cause other problems too. The heat can expand blood and speed things up too much. This can lead to headaches, poor and restless sleep, red face, irritability, anger, anxiety, loss of rational thinking and clear headedness, general uneasiness and feelings of discomfort, rashes, bleeding gums, bad breath and toothache. In extremes it can also lead to delirium, fever and haemorrhage. Again to counter this, we need to avoid hot and phlegm filled foods. And add in lots of cooling bitter juices, green tea and vegetables.

If heat combines with dryness. It can quickly deplete your fluids and blood. Leading to symptoms such as dry skin, constipation, tiredness and shortness of breath. In extremes it can cause exhaustion, fainting and delirium. Lots of cooling and moistening foods and fluids are needed here. Particularly ones like mango, orange juice, coconut, apple and banana. These will rebuild fluids and nutrients. Obviously, in this situation, drink plenty of water to quickly build fluids and raise blood levels. Once your condition has been stabilized, add in salty foods, which will also help to lock in moisture and nutrients.

The Summer Sun.

Too much sun, can of course lead to skin cancer. So avoid over exposure and getting burnt. It also causes wrinkles and can speed up aging of your skin.

This leads us to the most important thing about Summer. And that is to make sure you do get some sun exposure. Too many people these days stay indoors playing computer games or get stuck behind an office desk. While you can indeed get too much of it, you can also cause many ills by not getting enough of it. It revitalizes, heats and powers up our bodies and everything in them. It is a source of pure energy. Just as its power can be caught these days in solar panels, our bodies too can recharge our batteries from it. In Western terms, the sun's power is stored within us through Vitamin D. According to Western researchers we need only expose our faces and uncovered arms for about ten to fifteen minutes, four to five times a week, to start to create and store plenty of Vitamin D from the sun. You can get Vitamin D through some foods, such as liver, oily fish, eggs and sun dried mushrooms. But these doses are relatively small in comparison to what the sun can provide you with.

Researchers have linked low levels of Vitamin D with increased risk of Alzheimer's disease, Osteomalacia (softening of the bones), infections, colds, flu, heart disease, stroke and high blood pressure. Whereas high levels of Vitamin D in the body, have been linked to lower rates of colon, prostate and breast cancers.

Scientists at the Medical University of Graz in Austria found that the people with the lowest levels of Vitamin D in their study, were about twice as likely to die from any cause over the next eight years, than those with the highest levels. As reported in the Archives of Internal Medicine.

A team at the University of Warwick, looking at 28 studies on Vitamin D, involving 99,745 people, concluded that middle aged and elderly people with high levels of Vitamin D in their bloodstreams reduced their chances of getting heart disease by 43 percent.

Autumn.

The sun starts to distance itself from our position on the earth and we start to cool down again. The summer has left us plenty of food to store and keep us going through winter.

Sometimes in autumn we can be affected by wind and dryness. Dryness can lead to chapped lips, dry skin and hair, dry eyes and dry cough. As it penetrates and dries internally, it may lead to constipation. And to low mood if fluid has been depleted from our blood, and our minds are then deprived of it and the oxygen it contains. To boost fluids drink water, apple, mango and orange juices. And have plenty of neutral, sour and salty fluids. Foods that are oily, like nuts, seeds and olive oil will also help.

The wind can be a very dangerous element. It tends to increase and drive the other types of weather deeper into us. In summer it can push the heat against our skin, drying it out more quickly. Or with the cold in winter, it can push fresh cold against us constantly. Preventing our skin from having any chance to heat itself and quickly draining energy and life out from our bodies. Always try to avoid exposure to the wind and keep the body well wrapped up to protect against it.

In Conclusion.

Although we have discussed the elements in particular seasons, they can occur at any time. Sometimes this can be even more troubling as our bodies are unable to adjust quickly and can be caught off guard.

Our modern world has also created new problems. Between air conditioning, which can cause cool and chilly draughts which will deplete our energy. And central heating which can dry us out and use up our body fluids. To holidays which can allow us to go from one extreme environment to another, from a sunny climate to a cold or even snowy one. Our bodies cannot adjust to these changes so quickly, leaving us open to colds, flu, infections and many other problems.

So what can we do to protect ourselves ?

There are several main ways. Firstly through our clothing. We can wear lots of layers particularly in winter to keep our bodies at the right temperature. We can wear gloves, scarves, hats and whatever else it takes to keep our energy levels secured inside of us.

In general, we should eat foods that are warming in winter and cooling in summer. Drying in damp and humid conditions. And moistening in drying ones. Of course always give first preference to pre-existing conditions in your own system. For example, if you already have heat related conditions in winter, don't go piling in more spices, coffee and alcohol on top of them.

Lastly avoid doing too much physical, mental or any other type of draining work in any weather extreme. Keep the power in your body, where it can keep it working efficiently and protect you.

Section Seven - Sleep.

Chapter Forty - A Good Nights Sleep.

Sleep is another key to a healthy mind and body. It is essential for a whole host of reasons which we will consider soon. Without it we can quickly end up in a lot of trouble. We can start to make many mistakes. From poor performance in our work, to arguments in our relationships, and even dangerous driving in our cars. It is now believed that tiredness and sleepiness cause more car accidents and deaths in Europe than the total that comes from drink driving. The long term implications on the body and mind can be equally as severe. These include higher risks of many illnesses, including the worlds biggest killer, heart disease. To top it off, many people become grouchy, irritable and moody without that good nights rest.

Sleep provides the yin to the yang. It gives a balance between the heat, movement and activity of the day, to the calm, coolness and quiet of the night. It allows us to slow down and recharge.

We generally need lots of sleep when we are young and busy at growing our minds and bodies. We start as babies needing up to eighteen hours sleep a day. And this gradually drops to about seven or eight hours as adults. As we age further, we still need at least seven hours each night, but due to underlying problems, we often lose our ability to sleep well and end up getting less than what is required to keep us strong and healthy. It is now estimated that in the US, every other elderly person over seventy has some form of sleep disorder.

What's Going On When We Sleep ?

For starters, our adrenal glands and other hormones become quite active. In the first part of sleep, for about four hours, growth hormone is released into our bodies. This rebuilds, repairs and regenerates cells and tissues, as part of healing any damaged or ill areas, or just in general replacing and renewing of older cells into newer models.

The latter half of sleep tends to reduce growth hormone and increase another hormone, cortisol. Cortisol is often linked to stress in Western Medicine. As we encounter both serious and milder stress, our levels of it rise in the body. In Chinese Medicine, cortisol would be linked to our Jing Essence. It is being released into our bodies because we have somehow managed to create a short fall of the necessary energy, blood and other nutrients required to keep our systems running smoothly.

Because our bodies have evolved to follow a twenty four hour clock with nature, if the body is asleep and inactive, the hormonal system will start to produce and release growth hormone at around eleven pm. It is therefore essential to be in bed by this time. If you are still awake and active, your body will be deprived of the correct amounts of this hormone and you will age quicker and not be able to effectively regenerate your cells.

Another reason to be in bed early, is to do with the Chinese view of Yin and Yang times in the day. The Yang time starts when the sun is coming up and charging the particles in the air. This makes them more hot, active and busy. When the sun is going down the Yin time appears. The particles in the air begin to slow down, condense and become more cool. As you breathe this air in, it helps to slow things down in your body and mind which will allow you to enter a more deep, fulfilling and beneficial sleep. To calculate this time, find the midpoint of the dark hours of the night. Then make sure you are asleep in bed, about four hours before this midpoint. This way of sleeping fits in completely with nature, unlike our modern unhealthy schedules which are often based around television and work. Generally a safe time, to produce good healthy productive sleep is around ten pm. There is an old saying that "an hour of sleep before midnight is worth two after it". There is a lot of truth to that old wisdom.

Because of the creation and release of growth hormones around eleven pm in our bodies, and the cooler, more passive night time air and energy that we breathe in, you can start to see how damaging it is to try to stay up late or even work through the night. Night shifts can increase rates of serious illnesses. They have been linked to many conditions, including heart disease and cancer.

A study by the Institute of Cancer Epidemiology found that women who worked night shifts were one and a half times more likely to develop breast cancer than women who worked regular hours during the day. The International Agency for Research on Cancer, part of the United Nations World Health Organisation, now lists night shifts as a probable cause of cancer.

The next thing we need to be aware of about sleep, is that it has different phases that affect the mind. When we first fall asleep, we enter a light sleep for about twenty minutes. Which is then followed by Slow Wave Sleep. This is the deepest part of sleep. It is in it that the body tends to do most repairs and regeneration. The lower and subconscious parts of the brain tend to be in charge here. It lasts for about two hours. Next is REM sleep. This stands for rapid eye movement, because you can literally see the movement under the eyelids of someone sleeping. The frontal more conscious part of the brain is involved here. The sleep is much lighter and more dream like. And you can awaken out from it if you have disturbing thoughts. If however you stay asleep, you will return to slow wave and repeat the cycle three to four times over the night. Because the subconscious has already completed some of the work, each time you return to slow wave, you will stay there for a shorter time.

In Chinese Medicine, two organs are essential for controlling sleep. They are the liver and the heart. A strong heart helps to send the right amounts of blood, oxygen and energy to the mind, to help it calm itself and prepare for sleep. If the heart is unsteady or unable to do this, the mind may be left anxious and too wound up to turn itself off, keeping you awake and thinking. When the mind and heart have begun to quieten the body, the liver is said to pull excess blood from the mind and body into itself, which helps to turn unnecessarily active things off even further, allowing you to fall into a deep sleep. The liver often helps to regulate the bodies blood supply, giving more into our systems when we are exercising and active, and less when we are resting and sleeping. It can store up to 1500 ml of blood. It even helps to maintain a steady blood pressure by releasing blood into the blood vessels when required.

Chapter Forty One - The Benefits Of Sleeping Well.

Firstly, it slows and rests most parts of the body. This is typically seen in the heart by the decrease in the rate it beats at per minute. Obviously the heart and other organs can now run at reduced power. This allows them to gather strength for the next day and to preserve them in the long run.

Next it regenerates our cells through the use of growth hormones. This will give us our beauty sleep, keeping us younger and fresher looking, and slowing down our aging. It can keep our physiques and muscles more toned, fit and healthy. And both our organs and brains in peak conditions.

It also helps to allow our energy levels to recover. If we keep awake and running our systems for too long, we will burn our energy up. If we shut them down, we preserve our energy, it accumulates and recharges again.

When there is more energy in our environment we tend to need less sleep. That is why we need far less sleep in the summer when the sun is closer and providing us with an abundance of energy. And more sleep in the winter when we get less sunshine. Usually six to seven hours is enough in summer. And eight to nine does the job in winter.

Our other main source of energy is food. If we miss sleep, studies have shown that we tend to eat more calories the next day to try to compensate for our lower energy levels. This can lead to weight gain and its associated problems.

One study by a team at Columbia University showed that people who slept for 4 hours or less per night, were 73 percent more likely to be obese than those who got a full nights sleep. People who got 5 hours or less were 50 percent more likely and those who got 6 hours or less were 23 percent more likely.

Sleep repairs and helps us heal our bodies. During it our glands and hormones remain active, releasing essences to fix and rebuild any damage our systems have incurred. When we are ill or recovering from an accident our bodies need plenty of extra rest and sleep. This allows them the breathing space needed to carry out any essential repairs. Quite often the rest and extra sleep someone is forced to take during a hospital stay is actually playing a big part in their recovery. Their bodies are forced into becoming inactive and slowing down, which gives them the time and space needed for their own internal healing mechanisms to come to the forefront and take charge.

Sleep also helps to sort out the days problems. It gives our brains a chance to archive and organize our daily thoughts and memories. To clear some of the clutter from our conscious minds and to reset and refresh them, preparing them to start all over again the next day.

When the forebrain becomes active during REM sleep, it starts to dream, working through unresolved daily or past issues. In Chinese Medicine, our dreams can point to weaknesses in our organs. As we will see in later chapters, our organs when they are not working properly can cause emotional and mental problems in our minds. This is sometimes reflected in both images and emotions we may feel in our dream states. When our kidneys are not producing enough cortisol, adrenalin and other boosting hormones, we often feel fear in our dreams. The lungs too, if they are stifled and not succeeding in taking in enough oxygen may feel suffocated, producing threatening and scary dreams. Digestive problems and lack of nourishment in the body can make you dream of food and eating. When the liver overheats and fails to feed enough soothing blood into the tissues, you may begin to feel uptight and restless. When overly hot liver blood reaches the mind, it can cause it to become too active. Which can lead to irritability and even angry confrontational dreams. The heart too can impact on the mind leading to anxious dreams.

Of course if you have unresolved issues, past or present, these too will spill over into your dreams. This is often a cause of waking you up in the middle of the night. When your brain cannot resolve or get a handle on a problem, it becomes more and more active, until you eventually awaken. Other times it is successful in sorting and fixing a problem. And when you awaken the next day, you may find the answer and solution to something you had been searching for.

Finally, when we are well rested our bodies tend to work better. Producing lots of food and energy for our brains. This keeps us in a good, healthy and happy mood. Allowing us to easily cope and deal with any problems life throws at us. If we are tired, our issues can often seem to become bigger and bigger, as the brain fails to have the resources needed to think clearly and to solve problems. Our mood becomes lower and often swings, making us grouchy and irritable.

Chapter Forty Two   -   More Consequences Of Poor Sleep.

Sleep is a basic requirement and lack of it can lead to serious health complications over the short and long term. As energy decreases every part of your body starts to become affected and weakened, leading to an inability to function and eventually in some, to a physical or mental breakdown.

The mind can be severely affected. After a poor nights sleep, most people notice that they cannot think clearly to resolve problems. Their thoughts and memories can become confused and muddled. With extreme sleep deprivation, the brain can become overloaded with thoughts leading to hallucinations and even loss of reality. The mood too can swing and become erratic with increases in irritability and depression.

A study by scientists at the University of Michigan found that people with insomnia were about twice as likely to plan suicides or have suicidal thoughts in comparison to those who had no sleep difficulties.

Another study by Columbia University Medical Centre for the National Institutes of Health in the US, found that teenagers with poor sleep habits were 25 percent more likely to be depressed than those who had good quality sleep.

As sleep decreases energy levels will fall leading to weakness in the immune system, and the body will be left without enough power to create white cells when they are required to defend it from any invading pathogens.

A study in the journal Archives Of Internal Medicine by the Carnegie Mellon University, found that people who had less than seven hours sleep a night, had three times the risk of catching a cold when compared to those who had eight hours sleep.

The heart too can become overworked and badly affected by lack of sleep. A study by a team at the University of Chicago in the Archives Of Internal Medicine, showed that each hour of lost sleep increased the participants risk of high blood pressure by about 37 percent.

Another team at the Penn State University reported in the journal Sleep, that people who had insomnia for more than a year, and who had a short sleep time of less than five hours, were five times as likely to have high blood pressure, in comparison to those without insomnia who slept for more than six hours a night.

A study by scientists at Jichi Medical University reported in the journal of the American Medical Association's Archives Of Internal Medicine, concluded that chances of heart disease increased by 33 percent in people with hyper tension, who had less than seven and a half hours sleep nightly.

Another study published in the Archives Of Internal Medicine found that women who got five or less hours sleep were 39 percent more likely to develop heart disease, than those who slept for eight hours per night.

Cancer rates too increase with lack of sleep. A team of researchers at Tohoku University Graduate School Of Medicine reported in the British Journal Of Cancer, that women who slept six or less hours per night, had a 62 percent higher chance of breast cancer than those who slept for seven hours.

Chapter Forty Three   -   Sleep Problems And Their Solutions.

Heat.

Heat can be a big factor in causing sleep disturbance. From an overheated heart which cannot slow down the circulation in the body and the brain to cool and quiet it enough to enter sleep, to an overheated liver or stomach which may cause a wave of heat and activity during the night that wakes you up. Heat by its nature causes movement and stimulation of energy. Whereas at night, most of your body, your limbs, tissues, conscious mind, digestive organs and many others want the opposite. Even the organs that need to remain active will work at a slower pace, allowing them some rest to regain their strength.

All this inactivity reduces the bodies temperature. We are at our coolest at about five am in the morning. Obviously the rest of nature is doing the same, as the sun goes down, so does the earth become cool and still. Anything that therefore causes your body to heat up and become overactive is going directly against this. To get to sleep and stay soundly asleep, we must cool and calm ourselves through diet and other techniques.

A major cause of heat can come from eating late at night. As we now know, the stomach creates lots of heat and movement to break down food. This action, depending on the type of food, can go on for a short or a long time. If you eat at night then some of this movement and heat being generated can escape into the rest of the body, and in particular disturb the heart and liver blood.

As the hot blood enters the mind, it can over stimulate it, causing you to awaken.

Foods that are hot in nature are particularly problematic. Alcohol, spices, coffee, red or black tea and sugar can all cause too much activity in the body and mind leading to an inability to get to sleep or restless and disturbed sleep. Foods that are sticky, rich and create phlegm, like fatty meats and cakes, can block up the stomach and prevent it from cooling. To get around this problem simply stop eating at night.

However if you want, you can drink water or cooling teas like green and peppermint, or have a mildly bitter fruit or juice in the late evening. Their actions are all geared towards cooling and cleaning the stomach, which can help calm and settle it.

A rich, hot and toxic diet can cause major problems for our hearts and livers too. If we have too much fats in our blood, our hearts can become overactive and heat up, from having to push all this thickened blood around our bodies. Our livers which store blood and also have to help create bile to break down fats, can often overheat from the extra workload. Bitter juice and green tea at night and throughout the day will help to clean them and the rest of our systems, if they have become blocked by bad fats and phlegm.

A deficiency of cooling minerals and heavier particles can also throw your body off balance. This can lead to a surplus of heat, producing excess activity and poor sleep at night. To rectify this, you need to increase foods such as vegetables and seeds. These have high levels of minerals and over time they will build up in your body, cool you down and quieten your mind.

Another factor leading to heat at night, can come from stress. Stress tightens and obstructs the circulation, causing organs to have to rev up and push their way through all this constriction. The liver which performs hundreds of operations in the body, including trying to manage blood levels in the brain and the rest of the body, can easily start to overheat from stress. As it does this it heats the blood it is holding, then releases it. The hot blood eventually ends up in the mind, where thoughts begin to race and dreams can become more and more vivid, until they eventually wake you up.

The easiest way to recognize if heat is disturbing your sleep is simply to look for the presence of heat itself in you at night. Do you feel hot ? Do you have hot feet, hot hands, are you pushing them out of the bed covers and throwing blankets off your body ? Do you like to sleep with just a sheet to cover you, and the window open on a cold night ? Do you wake up feeling hot and sweaty ? Do you have heartburn or bad breath in the mornings ? Do you get bloodshot eyes, feelings of anger, irritability or frustration ? Does your mind race and over think, do you constantly toss and turn, searching for a cooler place in the bed and so forth. If heat is disturbing you, reduce your intake of hot and phlegm creating foods. Increase cooling minerals and bitter foods and fluids. These will cool you down and clear heat and toxins away.

Cold And Energy Deficiency.

If your body becomes too cold or your energy or blood becomes weak, the organs that control sleep, can lose their ability to function properly and to perform their necessary tasks. It seems an odd thing to say, but sometimes you can actually become too tired to be able to sleep. The heart and liver simply have not enough power left in them to get you off to sleep and to keep you in it. To remedy this you should boost general energy levels in the body and also blood levels as well. Blood can feed and nourish the organs, helping them to build their strength back up. Foods that are more neutral in flavour can be helpful for this. Such as white rice, eggs, nuts, seeds, raisins, chicken, fish and porridge oats. Add in a little sweet honey and a tiny taste of spice if your energy is very weak. And add extra water, vinegar, apple and a little salt with the other foods if your blood is really weak.

It is good to cool down at night, but if you are weak then make sure you keep your bedroom a little warm. A room that is too cold can itself prevent you from sleeping well. So make sure you have enough bed clothes and blankets to keep your body at a reasonable middle temperature.

Emotions.

A distressed mind or soul can keep thoughts active, making your sleep more dream disturbed and restless. Or it can even keep you awake and unable to fall asleep. By having a healthy body, good supplies of energy and blood, and good strong hormones, it will strengthen your minds ability to deal with life and limit the effect negative issues in your personal life are having on you. However, sometimes you will need to grow in your life and make real changes to resolve these issues. Refer to the later chapters on emotions for more help with this.

Modern Technology.

Science has created some leaps forward and technological advances that have provided us with a 24 hour society, filled with all sorts of gadgets and entertainments, but our bodies are still part of nature and are restricted to its rules. So although many advancements can be welcomed, we must become more choosy in fitting them into a healthy natural lifestyle, rather than allowing them to distort our rhythms and cause mental, emotional and physical ailments for us. It may be tempting to stay up late at night, watching television or using the internet, to go shopping at 3 am in a 24 hour supermarket, or take on some night shift work for the extra cash. But when we weigh these against the damage to our health and the future unhappiness that this will bring, we see a different picture. To stay healthy we should confine these activities to our natural active time, the day time.

Another problem we have developed in our world, is too much brightness. With all our street lighting and lights in city buildings, our darkness isn't so dark any more. Because of all this extra light we have created, it has even become hard to see the stars in the sky at night. If you go into the country, where there is not much artificial light, it becomes much easier to see the stars. What does all this mean for us ? Well that little bit of extra light disturbs our sleep and keeps our minds a little bit more active than they should be. We should, just like our ancestors did, have total darkness to sleep in. A simple way to accomplish this and too achieve a deeper more restful sleep, is to invest in blackout blinds or curtains for your bedroom windows.

Another modern technical nuisance is to fall asleep with a television set or some form of music player still running in the background. Although you may manage to fall off to sleep. You will not manage to achieve a good nourishing deep sleep. Your ears will still bring the noise into your head. If it is some form of negative sounds, for example from a crime show on the television, this can enter your subconscious mind and interfere with your dreams. Your are better off not watching this type of program, especially before sleeping. As the last thing that was registered in your brain, can be pulled into your sleep and disturb it. If you want to put something into your mind, then put something pleasant, serene or happy in there instead.

Over Sleeping.

Some Western studies have linked over sleeping, that is more than eight hours a night, as a cause of ill health. However, it is far more likely that your body is sick and unhealthy, and it is trying to get extra sleep in an effort to repair itself or gather and rebuild energy to deal with the real underlying problem. If you are constantly oversleeping, napping or requiring extra sleep, then you should check your general health and in particular your energy levels. To boost your energy, do breathing exercises and gentle exercises like walking, Qi Gong or Yoga. Eat more energy producing foods like white rice or mildly sweet and spicy foods. And get at least fifteen to twenty minutes of sunlight, several times per week.

If you have had your full nights rest, then after you have awoken be careful not too spend too long in bed drifting back into and out of sleep. Your liver has to release blood into your body to help wake you up and then pull it back into itself if you go back to sleep. If you keep doing this, you will waste the livers energy and may tire the organ out. It won't be able to function efficiently after that and may leave you feeling sluggish all day long.

Snoring And Sleep Apnoea.

Both of these are linked to fats and phlegm blocking up your lungs and head in Chinese Medicine. There may also be generally weak energy in the body and in particular in the lungs. You should immediately avoid all things dairy in nature. And also any other rich, phlegm creating foods. Eat plenty of white rice instead, it is good for drying dampness and phlegm in the body and also for providing lots of energy. If you are overweight, then losing fat will help your overall health and reopen air passageways in the lungs and head, allowing you to breathe more freely and with less noise.

Chapter Forty Four - Some Quick Tips For Good Sleep.

Develop a wind down routine for bed. Get into bed clothes and prepare yourself for sleep about half an hour before you go to bed. Do quietening and calming things. This will send signals to the brain that is time to start shutting things down.

If you are busy working on a creative project then sometimes thoughts will keep coming into your head, keeping you awake. Put a pen and paper by your bedside and use this to put your thoughts into. As soon as this is done you will find your mind is released from the cycle and it can start to switch off.

Keep your bed for sleeping in or making love in. Avoid using it for watching television or reading and so on. When your brain associates other things with your bed you may find it harder to relax in it and then have difficulty getting to sleep.

If you cannot get to sleep, then get up and drink a glass of cool water. The cold will deplete some of the energy from your stomach, heart and blood. This will cool down your mind, helping to turn it off and making you more tired in general.

Try to keep the same bed time every night, including weekends. If your mind gets use to this internal setting, it will very easily and automatically know to wind things down for that time.

Program your subconscious mind to quieten down, enter sleep and sleep deeply. This can be a very effective method. You will get details on how to program the subconscious mind later in the book.

Make sure you have a comfortable bed. It sounds obvious and simple, but many people sleep on their bed year after year without checking it. And as it becomes lumpy and deteriorates, so does their sleep.

If you feel stressed, frustrated and angry. Then massage your hands and feet using downward strokes away from your head and body. Then try pinching the tips of your fingers and toes. This will send hot energy and blood down and away from your head, allowing it to cool down and become calm. This technique can often help you fall asleep under those conditions but will usually take ten to fifteen minutes to drain the energy from your head, so be a little patient with it.

Make sure there is good ventilation in your room by leaving your bedroom door a little open or using a wall vent. You can also open a window if it is not too cold outside. When your room is stuffy it can cause you to overheat and can also weaken the good air and energy levels in the room and in your body. Without good energy the organs keeping you asleep won't function properly and may wake you up.

If you can't get to sleep, then don't lie there thinking over and over about not getting to sleep and the consequences that may cause you in your day tomorrow. This will only wind you up further, making it more difficult for you to settle down. The mind tends to create more of whatever it is thinking about. So the best thing to do is to think of something else or even to get up and do some relaxing or boring activity until the mind slows, calms and quietens down. Then you can try sleeping again.

Avoid arguing, over excitement or any other strong emotional states before going to bed. Avoid reading or watching anything that could also create these states. Things that distress and disturb your mind will have to be dealt with by your subconscious and conscious minds when you are asleep. These can easily lead to restless sleep, vivid dreams and nightmares or even wake you up.

If you are too hot or your mind is racing or overactive, increase levels of vegetables in your diet. Their minerals and heavier particles will cool and slow down the active energy, thus calming your heart and head. Beetroot and green leafy vegetables are quite good for cooling the blood and promoting sleep.

To treat sleep problems, always think of the bigger picture of your overall health in all areas, physical, mental and emotional. Concentrate on a generally healthier you and you will find that your sleep starts to improve alongside your overall well being.

Section Eight - Exercise.

Chapter Forty Five - Exercise.

There are three main categories regarding exercise that people usually fit into. Those who do very little or none at all, those who do moderate exercise and those who partake in strenuous exercise. Eastern traditions and culture strongly separate from the West on their views of exercise. They believe that doing too much exercise or doing more intense exercise like running and aerobics can be unhealthy for the body and mind. They feel that too much exercise uses up and weakens resources such as energy, nutrients and hormones in the body, taking them away from the organs that need them to stay strong and healthy.

For the last several thousand years the Chinese have been studying the effects of exercise on the body over peoples entire lifetimes, they see no difference between strenuous exercise and being overworked as a labourer on a farm, a soldier in the army, a coal miner or some other intensive form of work. Which can often drain the life out of an individual, eventually leading to more weaknesses and illnesses, premature aging and an early death.

However, in Asia they also believe that doing nothing at all is equally as bad as doing too much. So they advise to do moderate exercise. This gives you the good benefits of exercise without any of the problems caused by over exercising.

In the next series of chapters we will discuss the three types of physical activity, beginning with Western exercise.

Chapter Forty Six - Western Exercise.

There are different intensities of exercise in the West, from walking to running. For this part of the book we will concentrate more on the strenuous activities that are popular in the West, like running, aerobics and competitive sports. That is anything that gets your heart thumping, pulse racing or your lungs panting for more than a short period of time. Or that breaks you out into a strong sweat.

There are benefits you can get from intense exercise, such as increases in circulation and a reduced risk in cancer, but these can also be achieved by more moderate exercise. So the question becomes, should we really be doing hard intense exercises ? Well lets take a look at a few problems it can cause and see whether it is still worth it.

Firstly, It depletes your energy levels rapidly. You literally burn up your energy as you force yourself through whatever difficult activity you are doing. A little bit of activity can wake you up and get your energy to come alive, but when you keep pushing, your stores of energy soon start to be used up. In particular you use up levels of stored energy from the food you have consumed.

When your energy becomes weak, both the organs and the mind have less power to do their jobs, so the system starts to become weaker. This will literally have implications for the entire body and mind. Nowhere will escape. Every part of you, from the digestion, to the liver, to the kidneys, may all lose their energy and begin to weaken.

One such area is the immune system. As we have learned previously, anything that weakens your immune system, be it cold or now exercise, leaves it without any power to build an army of defender cells when your body comes under threat from external bugs.

Athletes are often more vulnerable to catching colds than those who do not exercise. Many of them can also suffer from chronic infections. In fact, sturdy muscular American footballers are much more likely to pick up M.R.S.A. than the general population. Many teams have to disinfect equipment regularly to try to combat this. However in reality their real threat has not come from exposure to gems on their equipment, but from draining the life force from their immune systems through over exercising.

Other organs like the heart can over time weaken from the loss of energy. Even in Western Medicine they understand the importance of the heart maintaining good power levels. They recognize that there is an electrical pulse that keeps your heart going. An artificial pacemaker provides electrical impulses to create this pulse if your heart fails to have enough power to do so. When you over exercise, you may weaken the electrical energy your heart needs to have to keep a strong and steady beat. This may be one of the causes of sudden cardiac death. A condition which causes seemingly healthy athletes to drop dead during intense exercise. Sudden cardiac arrest affects more than 400,000 people in the U.S. every year. According to the International Olympic Committee, it is estimated to kill anywhere from 1 in 15,000 to 1 in 50,000 athletes. That gives athletes about three times higher chances of suddenly dropping dead than an average ordinary person has.

The physical heart too, is often put under major pressure by extreme exercise. In some athletes, such as rowers and cyclists, the heart can increase its mass to nearly twice the size of a normal heart. Other conditions such as obesity and high blood pressure can cause the heart to enlarge as well, but unlike exercise these are clearly recognized as bad for you in the West.

Another sign of weakness in the heart in athletes is the slow pulse rate. In healthy energetic babies the pulse is around 160 beats per minute. As you age it slows down. In young adults it is about 80 beats per minute, in the elderly it can be as low as 50 to 60 beats per minute and in athletes only 40 to 50 beats per minute. In Western Medicine this is because athletes hearts are said to be working more efficiently. Perhaps they are or perhaps it is because their heart energy has weakened.

A study by St. Lukes Mid-America Institute looked at 781 college athletes using electrocardiograms, between the ages of 18 and 21 years old. It found signs of heart abnormalities in about one third of them. And found signs of potential heart disease in one in ten of them.

Another study from New York University appeared in the American Journal Of Cardiology. The study which focused on 17,000 men, found that those who exercised hard enough to break into a significant sweat five to seven days per week, increased their odds of atrial fibrillation by 20 percent. This was in comparison to those who did no vigorous exercising. This heart rhythm disorder can lead to fainting, heart attacks and strokes.

Exercise also depletes levels of nutrients in your body and in the blood itself. It does this in several ways. Firstly they are used up during the demands for energy from the exercise itself. Then after the exercise, blood and nutrients are used to repair damage to your muscles caused by the strenuous activity. This obviously has a detrimental effect on the rest of the body as well. The blood has now been depleted and weakened, so it is less effective. It is being directed to the large muscles found in the legs, arms, back and chest and away from the organs and the brain, which need it the most to keep everything running healthily. On the outside, the muscles are becoming bigger, more well defined and toned, but internally the organs are paying the price for this.

Another sign of blood deficiency appears in female athletes, the blood may become so weak, that periods can become irregular and even stop altogether.

The most serious consequence in Chinese Medicine from over exercising, is to do with depletion of the Jing essence in the body. This substance helps to create your hormones. Every time your body comes under any threat, the adrenal glands will release some of this substance in the form of hormones into your system. When you over exercise you usually end up tearing the muscle fibres. These will need to be rebuilt, so the body uses growth hormones and other ones to do this. This is why many body builders and athletes will often take cortisol, testosterone and other steroids to build extra muscle and power in their systems.

When you deplete your own natural hormones, the consequences of this are two fold. Firstly it directs these vital substances away from more important areas, which are your organs and your mind. And secondly if you persist in constantly demanding more and more hormones to repair and rebuild muscles, you may find that the adrenal glands and other important hormone creators eventually tire out. With this exhaustion they lose their power to even create the necessary hormones to run and keep the rest of the body healthy. Although physically the muscles may be toned, you might find in other ways the body becomes weaker and weaker. Later, in this book, we will look at the major problems created when the Jing essence has been over used.

The mind can also be badly affected by too much exercise. When levels of energy, blood, nutrients and hormones have fallen or have been redirected away from the brain, it begins to cause low moods, swings, anxiety and other mental illnesses. The short term affects of strenuous exercise can mislead and fool the athlete into thinking their mood is improving. They will initially get lots of oxygen pumped into the brain, which will give it a temporary high. And while their adrenal glands are still functioning properly, they will also get a boost from hormones released into the bloodstream and mind during exercise. However, as substances are used up and the organs weaken, then long term the opposite will start to happen in most people. And when they are not exercising, their blood, nutrient, energy and hormone levels will be lower than is required to keep their mind and emotions, steady, healthy and happy.

Other problems that can come about from too much exercise include the acceleration of aging. This can come from decreases in hormones and from depleting nourishing blood. And also from dehydration from intense activity and even from reducing body fat or oils to unhealthy low levels.

The Norwegian University Of Science And Technology, found in their study of 3000 women, that those who exercised daily or to the point of exhaustion had the highest levels of risk for infertility. As much as three times higher risk of infertility than the national average.

A study of 90,000 women by the University Of Southern Denmark, showed that those who played high impact sports like ball games, racket sports or jogging while in early pregnancy, had three and a half times more chance of miscarriage compared to those women who did no exercise at all.

Many studies have linked sports with arthritis and osteoporosis. The constant pounding and pressure on joints and bones is often too much to bare, leading frequently to problems in hips, knees, elbows, ankles, wrists, shoulders and spines in later life.

The Journal Of Occupational And Environmental Health reported on a Swedish study of 500 physical education teachers, it was found that they were more likely to have arthritis of the knee and three times more likely to have arthritis of the hip than the general public were.

A study at Coventry University interviewed 300 former footballers and found that 49 percent had been diagnosed with osteoarthritis. One in three had to have surgery since retiring from the game. And 15 percent of them were now officially registered as being disabled.

The British Journal Of Sports Medicine reported a study on 50 elite athletic swimmers. Nearly all of them had inflamed lung tissue.

Another study, this time in the European Respiratory Journal, also reported on a group of professional swimmers. They found that 70 percent of them, had airway hyper-responsiveness which can be a precursor to asthma. It is estimated that as many as one third of all professional swimmers have full blown asthma, 80 percent of which came about after they started swimming. The reason for this high level of asthma in swimmers has been blamed on the inhalation of the chemical chlorine used to keep pools clean.

However, high levels of asthma in athletes is not isolated just to swimming. A survey of 1,600 top athletes, conducted by the Norwegian University Of Sport And Physical Education found that approximately one in ten athletes, regardless of the type of sport, suffers from asthma or wheezing. Another survey by the U.S. Olympic Committee after the summer games in Atlanta, found that more than 16 percent of athletes responding to a questionnaire reported suffering from asthma.

In Chinese Medicine, the reason why professional swimmers in particular have such high rates of asthma is not just from the chlorine, but is because they are exercising to the point of exhaustion and at the same time breathing in lots of damp heavy air. At the end of their training session, their overworked lungs have no longer the energy to expel this damp moisture, which over time starts to weaken them and create breathing difficulties.

The history of intensive Western exercise is actually only a short one. Many gyms only began appearing and becoming popular on a wide scale in the mid nineteen eighties. There has not been enough studies conducted to see the long term effects of over exercising on peoples lives. However, with the understandings we can learn from the Chinese viewpoint and the emergence of many negative Western studies now coming to light, it is time for a complete rethink in the West. To move away from the promotion of hard core exercises to a more moderate version, which will be healthy and beneficial for everyone.

Chapter Forty Seven - Western Exercise And Weight Loss.

Something strange has happened in the West over the last few decades. Since gyms became popular, obesity levels have sky rocketed. It is claimed that exercise is great for weight loss, yet the results produced in our society seem to say the opposite.

A study by a team at the Louisiana University of 464 overweight women, who were assigned different levels of exercise for six months, found that the group who exercised the most did not lose significantly more weight than the other groups who did less. Another study by researchers at the University Of Leeds published in the Journal Of Public Health Nutrition came to similar conclusions.

So what's going on ? Well exercise certainly does burn up calories, but surprisingly not always that many. The average Westerner consumes about 2,500 calories a day. If you run for an entire hour you will only burn up about three hundred and fifty of them. This is not a huge amount in comparison to your overall daily intake. However with all this activity, you will also use up your energy and weaken your body. And this will inevitably cause you to become more hungry and eat more, putting the calories you lost through exercise back into your system.

The other side of this, is that with lower energy levels in your body, the rate at which everything else is running at inside of you starts to slow down. With less power your brain, kidneys, liver, heart, lungs and other organs, including the digestive ones will weaken and run less effectively. This will reduce the speed at which your body consumes and burns up your food, which in turn slows and limits your weight loss.

In 2007, after researching the subject, the American Heart Association and the American College Of Sports Medicine issued guidelines suggesting that in order to lose weight, they recommended people to exercise intensely for sixty to ninety minutes on most days of the week. Apart from what many would see as the torture of having to workout for ninety minutes and the impractical side of finding time to do that amount of exercise when you have a job, commitments and a life to lead, it also highlights how ineffective exercise is as a weight loss tool.

Finally if you do manage to reduce weight through strenuous exercise alone, you will also become tied and dependant on that method. If you stop exercising, the weight piles back on. Whereas if you make the right changes in your diet, the weight will stay off permanently.

For long term and permanent weight loss and also whole body health gains, a combination of good dietary practice and frequent gentle to moderate exercise seems to work the best and give the most benefit.

Chapter Forty Eight - Lack Of Exercise.

We have seen how doing too much can weaken, wear out and damage your body in many ways, but so too can a lack of movement and activity lead to many problems and illnesses. If you do nothing at all, organs start to become weak and things start to slow down and accumulate in the body. This can cause it to become blocked and stagnant on the inside. The heart and other organs will find it more difficult to do their jobs and will face a heavier workload and burden from this excess.

Whereas gentle movement and light exercises break up stagnation and encourage circulation. They squeeze and push vessels and organs, forcing things that are lying in them to be moved through. This stops phlegm and toxins gathering and adhering to cells where they can cause damage to them. This reduces the likelihood of many of our modern diseases such as cancer, diabetes and Alzheimer's.

Another pattern that can come about in the body from lack of activity is weakness. If muscles, tissues, bones, joints and organs aren't used, then energy is redirected away from them. Over time this will cause them to become weak and incapable when they are needed to perform an action. A moderate amount of movement will prevent this from happening.

One of the organs that can become affected by lack of movement is the digestive system. If it becomes sluggish and blocked, it will be unable to effectively digest and breakdown food which may leave you short of the good nutrients you need, but at the same time allow a surplus of damaging poorly digested ones into your body. These will create phlegm and fats in you. This extra weight can lead to even more problems and pressure on your already troubled body.

Chapter Forty Nine - The Right Type Of Exercise.

If you ever visit China, you will notice that the parks are filled with people in the early hours of the morning. In them you will see the people perform many different types of activities. Above all else they love to do moderate and gentle exercises. You won't see many sweaty and strained faces or puffing and panting individuals among the crowds. The Chinese exercise more frequently with less intensity. Spending thirty minutes to an hour doing more easy going, less strenuous movements.

These moderate activities do many things in the body, they help to move the circulation ridding phlegm and toxins from it. They tone and strengthen the muscles and make them more flexible and agile. They help to circulate blood, oxygen and hormones up into the brain, refreshing it and giving it a boost. They encourage the mind to focus on the movements, which can distract it, giving it a break from everyday anxieties and problems. The actions open the lungs, allowing them to rid waste and pull more oxygen into the body. They aid the digestion by helping to physically squeeze waste down through the intestines. They invigorate and stimulate the adrenal glands to produce a small amount of hormones into the blood stream. And they gently create, through the method of movement, more energy in the body.

The key factor to understand here is that these moderate exercises are giving you all the benefits of harder exercising without the drawbacks. They won't burn up and use up all your energy, leaving you tired and worn out after them. Or leave your organs weak and unable to function properly. Or your immune system left without power to build white cells if they are needed to defend you. And they won't leave your body and muscles damaged the next day, so there is no chance of these ripped tissues stealing and draining all your blood, nutrients and hormones away from your organs, where their use is far more beneficial and productive to your overall health.

As hormones and Jing are only needed in small amounts, these type of exercises won't over use or wear out your adrenal glands. The hormones released into your body will benefit the organs making them more efficient and strong and less likely to become ill. Over time this extra strength will reduce the overall demand for hormones caused by stress and disease. This will help to preserve your Jing for future use and a longer life.

They are also helpful and effective for losing weight, because they are creating extra energy through movement and breathing and not burning it all up. You will therefore end up with more energy in your system after you workout. This will increase the activity of all the organs. Giving them more power to effectively clean themselves of fats and phlegm and to generally become more productive. This extra activity uses up more calories throughout the day and helps you to regulate your weight.

Also because your energy is higher and your body is working more efficiently, you won't have cravings to eat so much food and this too will lower your calorie intake and reduce your weight.

The other big benefit of this style of exercise is that because it is simply less draining than intense exercise, you are more likely to stick with it and not be put off by the pain usually associated with the harder exercises. Moderate exercises are very easy to do and can be enjoyable and stimulating to both the mind and body.

The amount of exercise needed can change from one person to another. If you have an active job you need less. If however you have a sedentary job, like working behind a desk all day long, you obviously need more. If you are sick save your energy to treat the illness and don't exercise too much until you are on the road to recovery.

In general, about 60 minutes a day of moderate movement is a good level to aim for. This sounds like a lot, but it can be spread throughout your entire day and can include such things as brisk walking to work or to shops and so forth.

Try to make exercise fun and do as many things that you enjoy as possible, like walking, hiking, gentle cycling and dancing. You could put some music on and dance around for half an hour or go and join some dance classes. Also try leaving the car at home for short journeys. Try cycling to work if it's possible. And do simple things like, taking the stairs instead of the elevator. Parking the car at the furthest end of the car park, away from your destination. Getting off the bus a stop or two early and walking the rest of the way. Getting a pet dog, they will get you out for lots of walks and give you good company. And even mowing the lawn and general gardening can provide you with good exercise.

You can also simply, stand up in front of the television while you are watching a program and then step up and down on the spot for about thirty minutes. If it is a good program your mind will be engaged and you will hardly notice the time fly by, until your exercise is completed.

Tai Chi, Qi Gong and Yoga are great forms of exercise which will get you healthy but will also provide many extra benefits for the mind and spirit as well. If you wish to do more formal sports, try doing them in a more relaxed, easy going and fun way. Take the competition out of them. It will be better for your body and your mind and soul too.

There are now many Western studies appearing that prove how good moderate exercise can be for you. One such study was regarding Yoga. Researchers at the American College Of Sports Medicine found that a group of asthmatics reduced their severity and frequency of symptoms, and also improved their breathing and quality of life by more than 40 percent, by performing Yoga three times a week over a period of just ten weeks.

A review of 47 studies concerning Tai Chi, by the Tuffs New England Medical Centre appearing in the Archives Of Internal Medicine, found that improved cardiovascular and respiratory function appeared in both healthy subjects and patients practising Tai Chi. Some of the patients had undergone coronary artery bypass surgery, while others had heart failure or hypertension and some had suffered acute myocardial infarction. The studies also found benefits for arthritis, multiple sclerosis, pain, anxiety and stress.

The Honolulu Heart Study of 8000 men, reported its findings in the New England Journal Of Medicine. They found that walking just two miles a day, over a twelve year period, the length of their study, cut the risk of death almost in half. They found in particular that the risk of death from cancer was lower. Those who walked very little were two and a half times more likely to develop cancer, than those who walked the two miles per day.

A study by the University Of Michigan Medical School, of 9,611 adults, appearing in the journal Medicine And Science In Sports And Exercise, showed that those who were regularly active in their fifties and sixties, doing activities like gardening, walking, dancing and so forth. Were 35 percent less likely to die in the next eight years than those who were sedentary.

The Nurses Health Study reviewed information on 18,766 women between seventy and eighty one years old. It found that those who walked one and a half miles a week, had significantly less decline in their thinking abilities as they aged, in comparison to those who did no exercise.

The Honolulu-Asia Study found that men who walked two miles a day halved their risk of dementia, in comparison to those who walked less than a quarter of a mile per day. 2,257 men between seventy one and ninety three years old took part in the study.

Chapter Fifty - My Personal Experience Of Exercise.

At the age of thirteen I started practising martial arts. I began with Taekwondo, the Korean art famous for its high, jumping and spinning kicks. Four and a half years later, I went for and received my first black belt. At that time I trained intensely, doing as much as two or more hours a day five days a week. I began to have dizzy spells after some training sessions. So my Western medical doctor sent me to hospital for a series of tests. It was discovered that I had developed a soft systolic heart murmur, where extra muscle had developed in my heart and caused the flow of blood through it to become slightly irregular. I was put through electro cardiograms and many other tests. Their conclusion was that it had come from the exercise. And as at that time exercise was seen as being very good for you and there was less awareness of sudden cardiac death, their advice was to keep on doing it. So that is what I did. By my early twenties, I had added bodybuilding in with my martial arts routines. Physically from the outside I looked really well. My body was toned and muscled and gave the image of being very fit and healthy. And because of this outer impression I believed I was in top shape.

However after I began to learn Chinese Medicine and changed the intensity of my exercise routines, I was amazed to discover how unhealthy I had actually become from all that strenuous activity. Sure, I had the outward appearance of excellent health. But inwardly I had strained, stressed and weakened my body to the point of making it sick. My big muscles were literally draining away nourishment from my mind and organs, starving them of the essential substances they needed to be strong. The tiredness that I often felt, particularly on days of training, which I had simply put down to being a side effect of work from the exercise, was actually the life force being squandered from my body. Apart from this general tiredness, I often got colds and if I was injured or bruised it would take a long time to heal. But most troubling was the low depressing moods I would have and the swings in temperament. My mind too would be anxious and irrational at times. All of this came from it being starved of energy, blood, nutrients and hormones. My Jing essence had become weakened by such intense workouts that it took me years of right living and good practices to build it back up again.

I now fully adhere to the Chinese methods of proper exercise. I practice Qi Gong for at least thirty minutes daily. I walk in the fresh air and sunshine when I can. And I do practical and simple exercise routines to keep my circulation strong and active, and my muscles and appearance toned and shapely.

You can develop any routine that suits you. But for me, my own personal one is to practice Qi Gong daily. And also do a set of chin ups, bicep curls and press ups for about five minutes on one day. And on the next, I will spend five minutes simply walking up and down the stair case in my house. I usually manage about forty five to fifty lengths of stairs in this time. My breath increases but I don't puff and pant. My body gets warmer but I don't break out into a heavy sweat. And my heart beats faster but does not thump excessively in my chest. And most importantly, the next day my muscles are not left sore and aching, so I know my hormones and nutrients are not being squandered to repair them.

As I said earlier in the book, I was quite overweight as an infant and child. Exercise did help to lose some of that weight and was good for toning and shaping muscles, but the techniques I found through Chinese Medicine produced much more long lasting and impressive results. That were beneficial to my body, my mind and my spirit.

Section Nine - Jing, Sex And Aging

Chapter Fifty One - Jing.

There are three substances in the human being that the Chinese refer to as The Three Treasures. They are Qi, which is the very life force energy of the body. Shen, which is the mind and the spirit. And Jing, the substance responsible for our physical being.

Jing is the name the Chinese use for what they consider to be one of the most important substances in the body. It is passed on from the parents to the child during conception and pregnancy. The most comparable substances to Jing in Western terms are hormones, DNA and stem cells. Jing is in charge of producing sperm and creating a foetus in the womb. Of growing a baby to a child, a child to a teenager and a teenager to an adult. As it begins to run out we begin to age. When it has been exhausted, we die.

From a Western viewpoint our hormones are similar. They are in abundance as children, quickly growing our bones and bodies. At puberty there are more and different types like oestrogen and testosterone released into us to define our sexual characteristics and increase power and strength in our systems.

However, they don't stop there. Anytime we let ourselves weaken or come under threat, hormones like adrenalin and cortisol are released from our adrenal glands into our blood stream. This gives us a boost, gets us out of danger and heals us back to a healthy level. In middle and old age as our production of hormones starts to decline, there are insufficient levels of these hormones to keep us strong and healthy. Nor are there enough to rebuild and regenerate cells to the youthful levels they were before. Our Jing is simply running out.

A multitude of Western studies have shown the importance of hormones in keeping our bodies strong and powerful, and to how we increase our risk of diseases as they diminish in our systems.

One study of nearly 4000 men by a team at the University Of Western Australia and featured in the Archives Of General Psychiatry, showed that the participants with levels of testosterone in the lowest 20 percent were three times more likely to be depressed that those men who had levels of testosterone in the highest 20 percent.

Another study by scientists at the University Of California of 800 men over fifty years old, found that those with low levels of testosterone had a 33 percent increased risk of death over the next eighteen years in comparison to those with higher levels.

A group of researchers published a study in the journal Obstetrics And Gynaecology which reviewed the health outcome of 29,380 women from the Nurses Health Study. It compared women who had ovaries removed to those who had not. Ovaries produce and secrete oestrogen and progesterone. It found that many health risks increased for women who had their ovaries removed, such as the risk of heart disease which increased by 17 percent, the risk of lung cancer which increased by 26 percent, and the risk of death from any cause which increased by 12 percent.

A study of 43,277 men by a team at the University Of Southern Denmark, appearing in the American Journal Of Epidemiology assessed the health and life span of these men over a forty year period. They found that those with higher sperm concentration, those with 40 million per millilitre were 40 percent less likely to die than those with lower amounts of 10 million per millilitre during that period. Those with more active moving sperm, that is 75 percent of sperm had normal movement, had 54 percent less chance of dying than those with only 25 percent of sperm with normal movement. They also found that men with higher quality sperm had a reduced risk of many diseases, including cancer, lung and digestive diseases.

Time and time again Western studies and science have proven the power of hormones in the body. Their medicine often uses hormones to produce powerful effects in the body. From steroids used for the healing of injuries and general recovery from illness. To hormones used in fertility, lack of growth in children, delayed puberty, menopause and now even for rejuvenating men in old age.

Chapter Fifty Two - The Protection And Conservation Of Our Jing.

One of the foundations of Chinese medicine is the idea of Jing and its preservation. It believes that Jing is an expendable substance. If you use up too much too quickly, you will weaken your body, allow it to become more ill and shorten your life span. Whereas if you protect and don't overuse your Jing, it will provide you with a very long life of good health.

The kidneys and the adrenal glands, which are two small glands sitting on top of the kidneys, together with the reproductive organs are seen as the storehouse of your Jing. These organs can be seen like the roots of a tree in nature, which provide the real inner strength and health of the tree. If you damage the leaves, branches or bark, only those areas will suffer, and the main part of the tree will be left unharmed or can easily recover. But if you damage the roots, then the whole tree feels the effects and it may even die.

In the body, if you damage the kidneys or weaken their energy, then the adrenals will weaken too. This will weaken your production of hormones and the whole body and mind will be affected and left vulnerable. If they come under any form of threat, be it illness or stress, there will be no release of hormones and very little will be fixed and repaired. To the Chinese the most important aspect for your future health, is to have strong kidney energy and an abundant supply of powerful and healing Jing essence.

So how can we protect this vital substance ? How will we be able to have plenty of it left in our old age to slow down aging and increase our longevity, and to keep us strong and healthy and able to bounce back from any emergencies life throws at us ? Well firstly we need to examine what uses it up. The answer is simply everything that puts too much pressure on us and over stresses our minds and bodies. It is a really long list and includes such things as lack of or poor quality sleep, over working, drug use, dealing with a short or long term illness, and stress across all spectrums, from loneliness to aggravation, to anxiety and fear.

Fear in particular is noted with depleting power and essence from the kidneys very quickly. In Western Medicine it is understood that our adrenal glands will release lots of adrenalin into our bodies to cope with stress, but in particular the largest amounts will be released during times of shock. The adrenalin opens our minds so they can think clearly in a crisis, and boosts and steadies our hearts and blood pressure. It provides our bodies with the ability to enact the fight or flight response to a dangerous situation. To give us the power to take action and fight or the ability to run out of harms reach.

Other things that can deplete our Jing, are over exercising, starvation diets or even things like missing meals and shift work.

For men having too much sex and for women too many pregnancies too close together can also deplete Jing. This will be discussed in detail shortly.

Basically anything that your mind, energy and blood can't deal with by themselves will cause a demand for your kidneys and other glands to start producing hormones which will eat into your Jing. Once the Jing is gone, the Chinese believe it is very hard to get it back, so Chinese Medicine focuses on preserving it by keeping the bodies organs and mind functioning at their peak and keeping qi and blood at high levels. This way you end up using only the smallest amounts of Jing necessary to keep things running and in good health.

The most simple and basic rule to conserve our Jing is too avoid doing too much. Don't overwork or over exercise. Don't rush about or generally take on too many tasks. Avoid exhausting yourself and doing things too intensely. Instead take breaks and pace yourself. Do things in your own time.

To further strengthen our bodies and create less demand for Jing, we can make sure we get good quality sleep. Keep our minds positive and avoid stress. Learn and practice methods that allow it to protect and heal us, instead of relying on our Jing to do so. We should also eat nutritious foods that support our blood, energy, organs and in particular our kidneys. Bland and salty foods tend to be very effective here. They help to create lots of raw building blocks to renew and repair our cells and to generate fluids that act with our hormones. Salty foods in particular tend to benefit the kidneys and also help to lock in and astringe hormones into the body. Particularly noteworthy foods for Jing and kidneys are nuts such as walnuts, good plant oils, seeds such as pumpkin, eggs, goji berries mushrooms and cinnamon. We should also avoid too many heating and stimulating foods like coffee, alcohol and spices. These can overheat and burn up our reserves of nutrients, which can end up creating excessive demand for Jing.

All forms of recreational drugs like cocaine and heroin, and even some stimulating types of Western medical drugs are believed in Chinese Medicine to use up and quickly deplete Jing in the body. Leaving it in a weak state for future health.

However, the body seems to have a safety mechanism to ensure you don't use all your Jing at once. And if it is being demanded and depleted too quickly, then the body slows down its release to a trickle to preserve it. So if you have overused your Jing, then the downside of this is that if their aren't enough hormones being made to repair the body and keep it strong, you can start to get lots of problems.

In particular some of the following areas and symptoms may be created when we weaken our kidneys and Jing. Tiredness and exhaustion, weakness, lower back ache, sore knees and ankles, low will power, timidity, chronic anxiety, fear, nervousness, lack of strength, bad teeth and weak bones, premature aging, sexual dysfunction, lung problems like asthma and wheezing, fluid retention and swollen ankles. Weight gain, poor memory and mental health issues, incontinence and poor and slow recovery from most ills. In general you will feel worn out and as if you are running on empty.

Our kidney energy can weaken too. This means that we may have sufficient Jing but do not have enough power to turn it into useful and productive hormones in the body. This can come about from several ways. If we allow ourselves to become too cold then our energy will be depleted and the kidneys may not work properly. Particularly if we allow our lower back to become cold in winter. So make sure you always wear a good thermal vest and so on to protect it. Avoid too, ingesting too many cold or cooling foods which may pull the energy away from your kidneys and into your abdomen to aid with digestion. Add a little spice or even a little alcohol to your meals if you feel your digestive system is getting cold or powerless.

The last thing to consider in this section is lack of use of the kidneys, adrenals and other hormonal glands. If you don't use them regularly and do things like moderate exercise and controlled levels of sex, then glands are not stimulated and can eventually lose their strength and ability to produce their hormones. This may block off access to your remaining Jing, leading to your body being left unprotected and vulnerable to everyday stresses and sudden emergencies. With gentle stimulation of these glands through appropriate exercise and sex, they are maintained in good health and the small amounts of hormones released by them are kept in the body, stimulating and strengthening it. In the long term this will make it more robust and less likely to suffer from the ravages which may be caused by stress, illness and diseases. And so providing you with a longer, healthier life.

Chapter Fifty Three - Sex.

The physical act of sex releases energy and Jing into the human body. Its pumping action is like a piston building up energy and electrical charges until it explodes into orgasm, sending ripples and waves of energy through the body.

For women the physical side of sex is generally good and healthy for them. It gives exercise to the body, encourages circulation and creates lots of energy. If they are having sex with a male partner they will receive hormones from him and at the same time release a small amount of their own hormones into their systems. These hormones will strengthen and empower them. Making them mentally and physically healthier and more resistant to stress and disease.

For men however it is a different story. Although during the sex act they are creating hormones and energy, when they ejaculate they end up losing this power and those hormones as well. Generally the excitement and charge that was in men leading up to and during sex, disappears after ejaculation. Most men are left feeling physically tired and drained. Some can even suffer low moods shortly after. In general, if men ejaculate too frequently they can start to weaken their bodies. Their entire systems may become depleted affecting their organs, their minds and their emotions. They will find it harder to recover from illness and injury, and their overall health may become poor. All this can lead to premature aging and decline.

Because of this, Chinese Medicine recommends the following guidelines for men and sex.

1) In good health men can have more sex, but if the body is run down, weak or tired, then sex should be reduced in frequency.

2) Sex should be avoided during times of illness.

3) Sex should be reduced during cold weather and winter. As cold can deplete the bodies energy it can create a double effect on the loss of energy from the body after sex. Therefore men should always keep themselves as warm as they can after ejaculation.

4) Sex should be decreased with age. As men age their hormones and Jing naturally start to decline and run out in their bodies. Because of this, it is recommended that they slightly reduce frequency of sex after the age of thirty in order to preserve their Jing. As they get older through their forties, fifties, sixties and seventies, this frequency should be further reduced.

5) Men should continue to have the right amount of sex as they age and not avoid it altogether. If organs and glands aren't used they can become weak and lazy in the body. They may eventually reduce their output or stop working. If this happens, hormones may stop being produced and the body and mind will not be able to receive any of their benefits.

This last point also applies to women. Their hormone levels and general health can also be affected by a lack of sexual stimulation either with a partner or through masturbation.

For men the big problem with sex, is not the sex itself which is viewed as having many positive benefits, but the loss of hormones and energy through ejaculation. For this reason Taoist and Tantric sex have been promoted for their abilities to strengthen the body, mind and spirit. Taoist and Tantric methods encourage having fulfilling sex without always having to have the physical act of male ejaculation. This creates energy and hormones in the males body without wasting and losing them.

Traditionally Taoist men and women would use this system to feed their minds and spirits with the raw power created during sex. The extra energy and hormones created from it helped them live longer and have better health, giving them more time to cultivate spiritual energy for their after lives.

In Tantric and Taoist sex, it has always been very important for both partners to enjoy very satisfying and fulfilling sex. In order for it to be healthy and to create positive energy, both partners must be pleased, neither can be neglected. For this reason much time and thought has been historically devoted to sex in the East. Both the Kama Sutra and the Chinese Pillow Books detailing Taoist Bedroom Arts are examples of the study and effort put into developing this area.

Men in our Western society in order to promote their health can incorporate some of this philosophy into their own sex lives, by continuing to have sex regularly but avoiding ejaculation at the end of every act. They should limit themselves to ejaculating just once in every two or three acts of sex.

If men follow this method, they will have more hormones and energy in them giving them more vigour and life. And also very importantly, they will be preserving their Jing for their future health. If you are a man who does practice this method you will notice that anytime you don't ejaculate at the end of sex, your body feels so much stronger. Your energy and power levels are much higher. You are simply left more charged up.

Chapter Fifty Four -   Sexual Problems.

General problems regarding sex can stem from two different sources in the body. They can come from physical problems or mental and emotional issues.

Usually when they are purely physical causes the person will display general signs of poor health and often circulation problems as well. Improvements in their overall health can improve conditions like low libido in both sexes, which may be caused by a lack of hot active energy and hormones. Inability or difficulty in achieving female orgasm, which physically can be caused by lack of hot energy, low levels of hormones, and by poor circulation. And male erectile dysfunction, which may be caused by poor hormone production and obstructed or weak blood flow to the penis.

To help with these conditions and strengthen overall sexual health, common spices like turmeric and garlic, and small amounts of alcohol are good at warming and moving the circulation. Other foods like seeds, nuts, mushrooms and the spice cinnamon can build up Jing and hormonal fluids to help boost up the sexual organs. Moderate exercise can also strengthen the heart and increase circulation to the genitals. If bad fats, toxins and sugars are blocking the circulation, then the introduction of cranberry, pomegranate and green tea can help clear these unwelcome additions from the blood stream. Even tiredness can cause problems, so general good sleep, eating energy producing rice and avoiding stress and overwork can all help.

However in the case of male premature ejaculation, this disorder if arising from a physical cause, is usually the result of too much heat and not enough cooling substances. There is too much pressure and over activity in the sexual organs and glands so they must be slowed and cooled. Bitter fruits and juices such as cranberry will help to relieve excess and reduce pressure in the sexual organs. Cooling foods like vegetables and sea weeds will help gather minerals and pull excess heat and energy away, thus slowing down activity. Small amounts of salt will also cool and astringe hormonal fluids like semen. Whereas any foods that cause heat will speed up activity and generally increase this condition, such as coffee, alcohol, spices, sugar and too much red or black teas.

When it comes to mental and emotional problems, these can have just as big or even sometimes a bigger impact on sex in all ways, both physical and psychological. Our modern culture has caused many new problems in this area for us. Although it has led us to become more expressive about sex, it has also generally led to a cheapening of sex and love. This has created many unrealistic expectations regarding sex and relationships. Sex has been used through advertising to sell meaningless products and is constantly used in television programmes and movies just to add excitement, regardless of the emotions involved in the story lines. Rather than portraying sex in a natural healthy way, some members of the media have turned it more so into a Hollywood performance. When real sex fails to live up to these high expectations, it can lead to feelings of inadequacy amongst ordinary people. Sex is like everything else, for most people that means it takes practice, open communications and consideration between both partners before it can become something special and fulfilling.

Poor quality relations or abusive ones in the present or the past, can also lead to problems in the bedroom for both men and women. For many people, if they feel they are being used, demeaned or even unloved and rejected in any part of their relationship, physically or emotionally, it can cause psychological issues for them resulting in problems like erectile dysfunction in men and vaginismus in women. This is a condition where muscles subconsciously and involuntarily tighten around the vagina, making intercourse painful or penetration impossible. Past abusive relationships, feelings of guilt or shame, incorrect notions we have learnt from society about sex, or even disturbing thoughts and images which can play on the mind, can be dragged into our present relationships causing problems for ourselves and our partners.

Modern culture is also creating many psychological problems and encouraging poor choices for partners in our relationships. It is presenting only the most beautiful faces and toned bodies in mainstream television and movies. Most of these people were born pretty to start with. Many then spend hours exercising in the gym to create curves and muscles, and some resort to plastic surgery or botox to further enhance themselves and to hide away any natural signs of aging. Ordinary people simply cannot live up to these standards but are now unfortunately comparing themselves and their partners to them. So rather than working at their relationships and making the most of and enjoying what they have and can create, their minds instead have become fixated on achieving something unrealistic and unobtainable which inevitably leads them to disappointment, sadness and relationship difficulties.

Women are now also groomed by movies and modern media to avoid men who are regular, decent and hard working. To avoid the "nice guys" and instead to go after those with a so called exciting "bad boy" image. However real life is not like the fiction in movies and instead in reality these type of men usually only end up abusing and mistreating their partners, leading to years and in some cases decades of real suffering and often physical and psychological damage for them, and also for any children they may have in such a relationship.

A group of researchers from the University Of Pisa, found that hormones causing the initial rush of lust and excitement in a relationship only last for a year or two, then drop back down to normal amounts, as reported in Chemistry World.

More research from Enzo Emanuele and the University Of Pavia discovered that an initial burst and higher levels of stimulating Nerve Growth Factor also decreased after just a year or two into a relationship.

If it has now been shown scientifically that sexual chemistry and lust only lasts for a year or two, it is not surprising that so many modern relationships are falling apart so quickly after that initial lust period. People need to become more wise and start using their intelligence and deeper souls to choose their long term relationships. People need to look for things that are long lasting, such as honesty, sincerity and a willingness to put real effort into building and growing the relationship. All these are required, if it is to have any chance of succeeding and turning into a beautiful one that will bring happiness, joy, fulfilment and real love to both partners.

Chapter Fifty Five - Fertility.

In Chinese Medicine it is believed that the current health of the parents, both mother and father, is passed on at conception. Therefore in order to give the child the best chance at life it could have, both parents are encouraged to get themselves as healthy as possible, both physically and emotionally before creating a baby. It is believed that the act of conception too, should be performed in a loving, peaceful, happy and healthy environment. Sex for procreation should be avoided after excessive drinking, when partners are sick, run down, stressed, traumatized, overly tired and so on.

Infertility Problems.

Most male infertility problems, come from the presence of toxins in the lower body. This damages hormones and can rot sperm. If you have infertility issues and symptoms of heat and toxins, such as constant yellow urine which is not turning to a pale or clear shade at some point during the day, odour from the urine, constipation or odorous bowel movement, skin problems, bad breath, anxiety and irritability. Then you should drink and eat plenty of green tea, bitter fruits and juices, particularly cranberry and pomegranate. These will help to clean away toxins and heat from your reproductive area. You should also avoid consuming heating and phlegm producing foods such as fatty red meats, sugars, dairy, alcohol, spices and coffee. If you smoke or are overweight, then weight loss and giving up smoking will also benefit you and reduce heat and toxins in your body.

It is also very important to avoid external heat from hot tubs, baths, laptop computers, electric blankets, car seat warmers and so forth. These can lead to overheating and can damage the sperm. Tight fitting underwear can cramp the testicles leading to overheating as well, so wear loose fitting garments instead.

In a three year study by a team at the University Of California, reported in the Journal Of The Brazilian Society Of Urology, researchers found that the sperm counts in 5 of 11 men with fertility problems, increased by an amazing 491 percent after they stopped having hot baths and Jacuzzis. The movement of the sperm also increased from 12 to 34 percent. 5 of the 6 men who did not improve were chronic smokers. The researchers felt that this influenced the lack of response in these men.

Another study by Spanish researchers reported in the Journal Fertility And Sterility, found that of 61 men in the study, those with poor semen quality had higher intakes of processed meats and high fat dairy, whereas the men with normal sperm tended to consume less meat and dairy and instead have more fruit and vegetables.

If you have infertility issues and are rundown and tired, then you should try to strengthen sperm, Jing and hormones in general. Cut out any intense exercising, ease up on over working, and try to avoid as much stress as you can. Eat lots of nourishing foods, such as rice, nuts, seeds, eggs and mushrooms.

Female infertility can be much more difficult to treat. Exact patterns are complicated and would require an entire book dedicated just to themselves. However general improvements in overall health can be very beneficial and may just produce the desired outcome. So you should try to balance your body and bring it into as best general health as you can. Sometimes this is all you will need to do. But if you are still not successful, it may be better to approach a Chinese practitioner who can treat you and give you guidance as to the more finer changes you need to make in your lifestyle.

Stress is one issue that does seem to play a big part in many cases of female infertility. Making positive changes in your mind set can be a huge help. Advice on this and other mental and emotional adjustments, is given later in the book.

It can be a slow process to encourage fertility in the body. I have treated many couples for this condition. In my experience it has taken from as little as a month to as much as eighteen months of treatment, and co-operation and work on their side to make their lives more healthy, in order to achieve a successful outcome in most cases.

Pregnancy.

While sex and ejaculation can use up too much Jing and hormones in men, too many pregnancies, either miscarriage or full term pregnancy, can deplete the Jing essence in women. It is therefore advised to try to leave adequate space between pregnancies to allow hormones to be recuperated in a woman's body. The length of time required may be different from one woman to the next, it can be different depending on her constitution and other background factors. However, women should always strive to get their general health and strength back before attempting another pregnancy.

When a woman becomes pregnant, it is obviously advisable to avoid any hard or excessive work and stress, to eat healthily and avoid smoking. It has always been noted in Chinese Medicine and culture, that both physical and emotional aspects from the parents and from during the pregnancy are passed onto the child. Pregnant women have been traditionally advised to take care of their minds and emotions during this time. They have been told to avoid ugly scenes and instead immerse themselves in peace, calmness, joy, love and happiness. This is said to produce a content and loving child. And to give it the best start for a happy and creative life.

Many Western studies now seem to be backing up this idea. From studies concerning mothers who have recently become overweight and are passing on higher risks of weight problems to their children. To other studies regarding stressful emotions and trauma in pregnancy, which have led to children with more temperamental emotions, and psychological and physical diseases in later life.

A recent study carried out at Nagasaki University and reported in New Scientist magazine, found that babies in the womb actually picked up and reacted to emotions from their mothers as they watched happy or sad movie scenes. It was noted that, the babies in the womb moved significantly more as their mothers watched uplifting happy scenes and became more still and subdued as their mothers watched more sad and weepy moments.

A study by teams from the Royal Veterinary College and London's Wellcome Trust, reported in the Journal Of Psychology, found that rats who were fed junk food while pregnant and breastfeeding produced offspring with high levels of fat in their blood streams. This remained there even after adolescence. The animals also had a higher risk of diabetes even if they were fed a very healthy diet. It is expected that the effects seen in rats, because of a number of fundamental biological similarities, would be repeated in human offspring.

A study by scientists at the Imperial College London found that mothers who were stressed during pregnancy delivered children who had increased risks of a range of mental and behavioural problems, with a doubling of the risk of Attention Deficit Hyperactivity Disorder. Stress caused by rows with a partner or violence was found to be particularly damaging.

During pregnancy women should continue, as best they can to do gentle and mild exercise. When blood flow and circulation is kept strong there should be a milder and easier labour.

If there is significant blood loss during labour it can lead to symptoms like depression, mood swings, poor memory, confusion, anxiety, alopecia hair loss, pale complexion and dry skin. Chinese herbs can be very useful in treating these conditions and are often used by women in China after pregnancy to build their strength up again. If you do not have access to herbs, you can eat lots of nourishing energy, blood and hormone supporting foods instead. Such as white rice, raisins, nuts, seeds, good oils, fish, eggs, chicken, mushrooms and small amounts of salt, cinnamon and honey. You should reduce clearing and detoxifying bitter foods during this time in order to retain nutrients and hormones, unless you have signs of heat and toxins in your system.

In China, the month after giving birth is referred to as the Golden Month. During this time, women still have plenty of hormones running through their bodies. These had been focused on building the baby but are now freed up to support the new mother. If the mother has to return to work or housework too soon these precious hormones and Jing will be squandered. But if she can rest these hormones may do wonders for her health. They have been known to cure many ailments and weak conditions that had previously existed in the woman prior to the pregnancy. In China, friends and family often cook and clean during this Golden Month, leaving the woman to sleep, rest and be comfortable and warm. This allows her to build her mind and body up to vibrant health. For Western women, if they have responsible and loving partners and understanding families, it is a really good idea and very productive for their general health if they can follow this routine.

Breast feeding is considered to be very important for the health of the baby in Chinese Medicine. It is producing natural and purpose built nutrients designed especially for babies. It is the perfect food for them and is being delivered at the right temperature. The Chinese prefer to feed at regular patterns and not on demand. They try not to over feed which can block up the babies digestion, leading to an accumulation of toxins which can often produce symptoms such as irritability and rashes. Breastfeeding is also very important in helping to establish a connection between mother and child. Gentle massage is another way to bond with the baby and improve its health. This can obviously be very helpful in allowing fathers to connect with their newborn.

Chapter Fifty Six   -   The Cosmetics And Beauty Industry.

Our modern world running on capitalism and competition seems to be leading us astray. Rather than making our lives more easy going, comfortable, happy and healthy. It seems instead to be focused on destroying us in many ways. Our spirits, minds and bodies have all taken a battering. One of the ways it has found to damage us is through our self image.

Irresponsible members of the media, television, Hollywood, and the advertising and fashion industries have bombarded our minds with unnatural, unrealistic and unobtainable desires of perfect bodies. It started with simple things, like instead of using a genuine representation of us ordinary people, they hand picked the most attractive and beautiful people to be on television and in advertising. This further progressed to the airbrushing of these beautiful people in images in magazines. And even other things like the use of make up on men to enhance their features in movies and on television.

Another example of this manipulation is in the way many advertisements for beauty products will take someone who was born with a natural gift of glossy hair or beautiful skin, and then try to imply and pass off to us that it was the advertised product that somehow created this beauty.

But now this industry has taken an even more dangerous step further. With the emergence of digital technology these already pretty models and actors are not just having minor blemishes, such as acne and moles removed from images, but retouchers are also being routinely requested by advertisers to straighten teeth, add in hairlines, enlarge eyes and even lengthen legs and trim waists on already skinny and tall models. It has now become physically impossible to actually obtain the standards being set in these digitally manipulated advertisements. Everything has become fake, nothing is real anymore.

All this trickery is leading to serious psychological problems. From feelings of hopelessness and inadequacy, to rejection of our natural and real bodies, to stress and mental tiredness from constantly trying to keep up with the latest trends. It is even leading for some to increases in life threatening conditions such as bulimia and anorexia. And in boys and men, to massive increases in the use of potentially lethal and damaging anabolic steroids.

Most worrisome is the effect this is having on children and teenagers, many of whom have now very negative views of their own perfectly normal and natural bodies. Recent market research from America has found that over 40 percent of six to nine year old girls are now using lipstick and cosmetics outside of play situations to try to improve their own self image. You can be sure that many of these girls will grow up with feelings of inferiority and complexes about their appearances, which will no doubt burden, affect and sadden them throughout their lives.
The only way around these artificial sales tactics being used by certain members of the media and

advertising industries is to raise awareness in yourself and others to demand higher and more honest standards from them. In the event that that fails, which is probably highly likely, we must strengthen and bring clarity to our own minds, which will allow us to see through these and other manipulations in life. And will give us the space we need to concentrate on the real important and valuable things such as health and happiness.

One industry that thrives off making us feel bad and negative about ourselves is the very profitable cosmetic industry. Now there are some in this industry who do a very wonderful job, they help individuals who may have been in accidents and left with deformities, or others who may have been born with real physical problems and who have had to lead very difficult and sad lives. If a cosmetic surgeon can help improve their appearance helping them to lead normal lives then that is a very good thing. It is following the true spirit of medicine which is supposed to be helping people and enhancing their well being.

However there are many opportunistic surgeons who are now preying on peoples lack of self confidence and low self image. Most of these people are perfectly normal and fine. Their problem is not coming from an abnormal body feature but from a mind that has been harassed and fed negative self imagery. This negativity often comes from the very industry they have now turned to. Medicine is supposed to be about helping people and not about making them feel insecure and bad about themselves. If these lonely people are to achieve genuine peace and happiness, they will only find this by looking at and working out internal issues and not by changing their outward appearance.

The darker side of cosmetic surgery is the dangerous risks that can be associated with it, with death being amongst them. There are also the long term side effects that may appear from these procedures. Many people have been inadequately informed of future problems which may result from these operations.

TV programs have often widely exaggerated and misinformed us about cosmetic surgery. They have generated many unrealistic expectations about the speed and ease of changing body features. They regularly hand pick a few individuals who have had the most dramatic changes in their appearances. This exaggerates the rates of positive outcomes and fails to provide an honest, clear picture of the real results an average person can expect to achieve. It also fails to represent all the infections, complications and botched procedures which now seem to becoming more and more common. These programs seem to simplify and glamorize the operations, lulling the viewer into a false sense of security that everything will go perfectly and ignoring or glossing over the negative and potentially serious problems that may result from them.

Instead of being anti-aging, it now looks as if in the long term some of these procedures may have caused damage that does the opposite and actually speeds up aging. One of the problems stems from the fact that the body is very complex. You have over 50,000 miles of blood vessels inside you. After you have taken a scalpel to these it is impossible to attach them all back up again. This means that anywhere you have had surgery, there will be a diminished blood, oxygen and nutrients supply to that area. And with less nourishment this area tends to age more rapidly. In the case of a face lift all the intricate blood vessels can't be rejoined properly, this disrupts circulation to the face and may make you age quicker than if you didn't have surgery in the first place. It can also cause hair loss at the front and sides of the scalp from lack of blood supply.

After liposuction, where fat cells and blood vessels have been ripped and sucked out of the body. Some are now finding years later, that the skin in the area becomes rough, discoloured and loose. On top of that, because fat cells have been removed from that area, fat is collecting in adjoining areas and may cause unnatural looking lumps and bumps.

In fact, to counter these problems a whole new Western medical industry has developed to treat the mistakes and problems that are now coming to light from the cosmetic surgery trade.

Another cosmetic procedure which is beginning to be questioned is the use of porcelain veneers. To apply these fake white veneers, perfectly healthy teeth have to be sanded down in order for the veneers to stick to them. The lifespan of a veneer is only around ten to twelve years. When it chips or falls off the tooth has to be sanded down again for a new veneer to be applied. The problem comes when you try to repeat this a third time. Most often there is not enough tooth left to be sanded again, leaving you this time with the only option of having it replaced entirely by a crown or false tooth instead. Your once perfectly good tooth has now been destroyed, and has left you with a lifetime of high costs and painful dental treatment and recovery.

Even botox may create future appearance problems. Apart from the unknown long term side effects, it has been reported that muscles on the face surrounding areas where botox has been used, now appear to be over compensating for the unmovable areas. This means that they may create new frowns and crease lines in these areas, which may lead to more wrinkles in them. Under natural conditions without botox, these would never have originated.

Another disturbing element coming into play, is the alarming number of chemicals being used in the human body. A recent poll of over 2000 women in the UK, found that the average British woman, through the use of perfumes, lipsticks, deodorants, moisturisers and make up, is now applying over 500 different chemicals to her body every day.

It is inevitable that some of these chemicals must be having a negative and detrimental effect on the human being and the environment. For example, artificial chemicals found in some deodorant sprays have been linked to higher incidents of breast cancer in women. There have also been deaths from over exposure to fumes from deodorants in confined areas. If you are using one then be sure to use it in a well ventilated area. Or even better, try some of the new all natural, chemical free deodorants made from minerals that are now becoming more widely available.

Chapter Fifty Seven - Natural Beauty.

Real beauty comes from both the inside and the outside. When someone has an engaging, alive and charismatic personality, combined with genuine kindness and caring. Someone who embraces life and has a smile for everyone. Then this regardless of their age, creates real attractiveness.

However on the other hand, if you have the most physically beautiful person, but they are cold, selfish and shallow, then all desire for them is truly lost. So remember if you want true beauty don't just work on the outside but build love and happiness into your mind and soul as well.

In Chinese Medicine to work on the outside, we also have to work on the inside, but this time we are referring to our physical organs. For these provide our skin, nails, hair and complexion with all the nutrients, hormones and energy they need to keep them young, fresh and vibrant. They even help to give sparkle to our eyes. To help our organs it comes back to the simple principle of strengthening our general health, through such things as good diet, sleep, moderate exercise and good mental and emotional well being.

Gentle and moderate exercises can be very helpful in keeping us younger, giving us an attractive appearance and providing good circulation to our skin, hair and face. But be careful not to overdo it, more is not better, it will drain our nutrients, energy and weaken our hormones, especially in the long term. Qi Gong and Yoga are particularly useful in slowing down ageing by encouraging high levels of energy in the body and preventing our hormones from being used up. They will also help us deal with stress and through their breathing techniques, help us to cleanse the blood of toxins. The other obvious benefit exercise can provide us with, is its ability to help tone and shape our muscles.

As most of our regeneration of cells take place when we are asleep, it is obviously very important to get the best possible sleep you can. Getting to bed early before 11pm is essential. As the kidneys start to manufacture important regenerative hormones at this time and if you are still awake and active you will lose out on some of these.

Massage can be very beneficial to problem areas which seem to need extra attention. Gentle movements and also tapping and lightly patting these places can encourage circulation into them. Over time, extra blood and energy flow into these areas will build up and improve, giving a more healthy, toned and vibrant look.

Controlling emotions and remaining positive and happy is important too. Stress, irritability, anger, worry, sadness, hatred, jealousy and other negative emotions will deplete your energy, nutrients and hormones rapidly, creating wrinkles and accelerating your aging. Stress will cause tension throughout the body, muscles and skin, which will also encourage the emergence of new wrinkles.

In terms of diet, it has obviously a major role to play in keeping the body in good shape. For starters it can help cleanse impurities from the body. This can be achieved through the use of bitter green tea, fruit and juices. When the body is clean, we can reduce our consumption of these bitter detoxifying agents and then fill it with good plant oils, nuts and seeds which will help boost hormones and also moisten, lubricate and nourish the skin, nails and hair. We should also eat vegetables which will provide minerals and particles to cool, moisten and preserve the skin. White rice which will give energy to digest the vegetables and to power up our organs to provide good Qi and blood to our complexion. And small amounts of garlic, turmeric and plenty of peppermint tea to encourage circulation and movement of blood around our bodies and to the skin and hair.

Finally there are several things that we should avoid. As we know, cold slows down, congeals, thickens and preserves substances, just like are cool fridges preserve food. Whereas heat does the opposite. It speeds up and accelerates, it can burn and dry out moisture.

Now to have a certain amount of heat in us is very important, as it produces lots of energy, which helps to keep our organs active, alive and producing all that they should do for our minds and bodies. But if we start to overheat we upset the balance, we start to burn up and waste nutrients, leaving less than is required to keep us moist and fed. And in terms of aging we start to damage our cells. So in order to stay young and have a healthy glowing well nourished outward appearance we should make sure we are not taking in excessive alcohol, coffee, red tea and spices.

We should also avoid any overextended periods in the sun which can cook, dry and redden our skin. And also if we smoke then we should quit, smoking has been proven in many Western studies to significantly age the skin and body.

One other area to avoid is foods that create toxins such as sugars, fats and dairy. As they can also generate heat in the body and may lead to acne and other skin and complexion problems.

Chapter Fifty Eight - Choices.

When it comes to aging we have a few choices in the West. We can believe in the hype and propaganda by certain members of the health and technology industries. They promise us everything, from cures for cancer, to growing spare replacement body parts and organs, to living to 150 while we remain in a youthful body. But so far they have failed to deliver on anything even close. Most ideas they come up with seem to eventually become unworkable or have to be stopped because of serious side effects. Perhaps in the distant future they will make a breakthrough here or there, or perhaps they won't. But based on their past performance, it appears to be a big gamble to put responsibility for your future into their hands.

We are often informed that Western Medicine is making us live longer, but this too is often misleading and playing with statistics. What has happened is that the age of life expectancy is calculated by taking an average from the population of a country. Because great progress has been made not in increasing the actual length of peoples lives but instead in preventing death in the first five years of life, this has made the average life span seem as if it has shot upwards. For example according to the National Health Services figures in the United Kingdom, infant mortality rates, that is deaths per 1000 live births, reduced from 34 in 1948 to a mere 5 in 2006 in England and Wales. While in Scotland the figures went from 45 down to 5 and in Northern Ireland from 48 deaths per 1000 down to 5.

Another big factor which has lengthened peoples lives, comes simply from the numbers of people who have quit smoking. A staggering 65 percent of the male population in the UK smoked in 1948. This has reduced to a mere 23 percent in 2006. With women it reduced from 41 percent in 1948 down to 22 percent in 2006. Similar reductions appear across most Western countries. This has obviously had a dramatic impact in reducing premature deaths from lung and other cancers, heart disease and many other ills.

With these factors and other reductions in deaths in children from effective treatments for diarrhoea, malaria and other infectious diseases. And with better general hygiene, safety and health regulations, sanitation, cleaner water and basic improvements in heating, housing and shelter, the average lifespan figures have moved upwards. But in reality they have not actually substantially added many real years onto the end of peoples lives as claimed by some.

The existence the elderly currently face in the West is a grim one. Whether you are rich or poor, you are not immune to disease. And without a doubt rates of diseases and illnesses are sharply increasing in the West. The modern Western vision of old age presented to us seems to be that you should expect to get many illnesses as you age. Cancer, heart disease, dementia, diabetes and so forth. The Western picture painted is that you will suffer, becoming sicker, weaker and more frail until you die. Becoming arthritic, immobile, incontinent, dependant on others, incapable of caring for yourself and losing your sight, hearing and mental faculties. If you are lucky you get to stay at home, if not you are shipped off to live in an elderly care facility, where you may end up having to sell your house, belongings and spend all your savings on its high costs.

A poll conducted in England in 2008 which questioned 1001 elderly people over the age of 65 for the charity Help The Aged, revealed that 53 percent of them felt that age discrimination had become a common part of their everyday lives. And that 29 percent of them believed that health professionals tended to treat older people as a nuisance.

In 2008 a report by the Liberal Democrats political party in England, found that over 22,000 elderly residents in nursing homes and an estimated further 32,000 elderly in residential homes are being given dangerous drugs that they do not need. It is believed that this is solely for the purpose of keeping them sedated and more manageable, to make life easier for the staff in these care facilities.

The following year, a UK government review, found that the actual figure was closer to 180,000 elderly people being prescribed these anti-psychotic drugs. Of that figure they estimated only 36,000 should actually have been taking them. More alarming, was the fact that these powerful drugs are strongly linked to deaths in one percent of those who are on them. This means they are causing about 1,800 needless deaths in the UK each year.

It is an insane society that we have developed to accept and normalize such a fate for our older years. Instead of promoting love and responsibility, of taking care of our elders, our families and friends, society is pushing us to become hedonistic, to be selfish, to just care about popularity, excitement and instant gratification at all times. Leaving the moral issue of this aside, it is a very illogical and foolish stance to promote. The consequences of this recklessness causes everyone to eventually suffer. In terms of aging, when we breed a society that abandons and neglects its elderly, we will find that as we age, we too will endure a similar fate.

Until recently in China, India and most of Asia, the elderly having lived through and learned from many life experiences were seen to be full of wisdom and understanding, they were respected and appreciated for this. You would have whole families from grandchildren to great grandparents living together, socializing and helping each other. But like Western diet, Western culture has also started to infringe on Asian lifestyles. This has led to many young people heading off to work in big cities and to the break up of families in the process, thus leading to more isolation, mental stress and loneliness. It is by no small coincidence that the rates of illness in China and India are beginning to soar as they have adopted our Western culture and diet.

So if we stand by and do nothing, it appears that this isolation, ill health and suffering is what most of us can expect to have ahead of us. Unless however, we decide to take responsibility of our own welfare. If we decide to get healthy, properly manage our lives and make a big investment in our future health and happiness, then this bleak and hopeless vision does not have to be the way we end up our lives.

Chinese Medicine believes that if maintained well, the body should provide one hundred years or more of good health in all aspects. We should have active alert minds, strong mobile disease free bodies and engaged, content and joyful spirits until we pass to the next world. There is plenty of evidence to suggest that this is not only possible, but it is what most of us should be achieving.

If we get healthy and make the right changes now then we won't just protect our futures but we will also feel good and start to see the rewards of our efforts in our present day lives.

Chapter Fifty Nine - What We Can Do To Slow Down Aging ?

Well Let's Start With What We Need To Avoid.

Smoking tops the list. Not only will it speed up the aging of your cells, but it will dramatically increase your risk of dying prematurely and often painfully, from diseases like cancer, lung failure, heart disease and many others.

Next up we have anything that causes too much heat and stimulation. This includes too much sun, alcohol, spices, coffee and indirectly sugars and fats. Any stimulant in excess will start to burn up and feed off the nutrients in your body, in much the same way as petrol or alcohol poured onto a fire will burn the logs up too quickly and quench its life.

Recreational drugs like cocaine and heroin, and Western drugs that act like stimulants can also fit into this category. In Chinese Medicine they are seen to give you a high or pain relief and so on, by releasing your Jing and hormones into your blood stream. Where in, dependent on your choice of drug, it may be directed into the muscles and organs to heal and build them or into the brain to give it a high.

After this we must avoid squandering our Jing and hormones. Basically this means that you need to adjust your life, to avoid work and play that exhausts you, leaving you feeling drained and wiped out. And of course for men, they should avoid too much ejaculatory style sex, particularly as they age into middle and senior years. By keeping ourselves generally healthy and avoiding over doing things, we will preserve our Jing and hormones for a longer period and extend our lives.

We have already previously discussed many of the things to do to increase our present well being. All of these of course will help to build up reserves, Qi and strength which will also slow down aging. So we will look at just a brief description of each one below.

Moderate exercise will help to keep muscles and organs in use. It will move your circulation and help clean your blood and other parts of your body in the process. It will help to stimulate your parts, stopping them from seizing up or gathering toxins that lead to blockages and damages.

Other exercises like Qi Gong, Tai Chi and Yoga are very beneficial in multiple ways to slow down the process of aging. These will be discussed in detail later.

Proper breathing and posture helps rid the body of toxins which may damage and rot cells. And therefore prevent the call for increased usage of your precious hormones. It also floods your body with energy producing oxygen to keep you powered up. In particular it powers your immune system with energy to help keep you defended and stronger.

Sleep provides the rest your body needs to slow down, keep itself cool and therefore not burn itself up and accelerate aging. The more rest you get, the better chance the body has of keeping itself healthy. If you don't get enough sleep you will start to overuse your hormones and weaken them.

We have already discussed avoiding too many stimulants and heating foods, as they speed things up and escalate aging. The opposite of this is obviously foods that cool and calm, they will benefit us by slowing things down. In particular, foods with minerals and heavy cooling particles will help to do this. Such as our fruit, vegetables, nuts, beans and seeds. Many studies are now showing us that traditional plant based diets, such as the Chinese and Mediterranean diets, can not only keep us healthier but can increase our longevity, whereas those who consume lots of meat and dairy tend to have more general ill health and a shorter life span.

Too much sun can burn us and speed up aging, but without it we won't get the benefit from its energy or create Vitamin D in our bodies. So 15 to 20 minutes exposure four or five times a week will help keep us charged up. We also need to have respect for the other elements, the cold, wind, damp and dryness. As over exposure to these can weaken our systems and their resources.

Next we have emotions. It is obvious that too many of the wrong kind, that is negative ones, can quickly make our minds and bodies sick and unhealthy. In the long term this can have a devastating impact on us, not only wasting our Jing and hormones through the release of cortisol, adrenalin and other hormones, but also impacting on our hearts and other organs. Those bad emotions simply weigh us down and inevitably wear us out.

Another factor that can affect aging and comes from the mind is our perception. If we listen to the media and culture without questioning them, then we will be deluged by an onslaught of negativity towards aging. The TV and movies now often portray the elderly as needy, useless, grumpy and unproductive. Disease has become so commonplace that it is nearly becoming an excepted and normal part of peoples lives. If we give into these perceptions, then our minds will start to subconsciously create and portray these events in our own lives. If we challenge them and teach ourselves methods to reprogram our minds, such as positive thinking and meditation, then we can alter this garbage being fed to us. This will not just prevent it from having a damaging impact but will also allow us to replace it with a brighter and more positive stance, which will protect us and keep us healthy on the inside. When we are faced with negativity surrounding aging, reverse it and instead bring your attention to youthful ways. Focus your mind and intention on staying young, mobile, fit, healthy and happy.

The mind is like the muscles in the body, if you neglect its use it begins to lose strength and weaken. So keep your mind active and interested. Particularly if you retire from work, don't just sit around doing nothing, instead keep learning, reading books, keeping it interested, motivated and enthusiastic. If you give up on these things, processes in your brain will begin to shut down and fade away, never to return.

A study by a team at the University Of Pittsburgh presented at the American Psychosomatic Society's annual meeting, found that women who reported themselves to be optimistic were less likely to die of any cause, and had a 30 percent lower rate of heart disease, whereas women scoring high on hostility and stress scores had a higher general death rate and also 23 percent higher rate of dying from cancer by the end of the study. The research was based on the personality traits of 100,000 women in the Women's Health Initiative Study run by the National Institutes Of Health.

Another study appearing in the Journal Of Personality And Social Psychology of 660 people, found that those with positive perceptions of their own aging outlived those with more negative views by an average of seven and a half years.

Finally, remember that aging is a natural and healthy part of the journey of life and the soul, that God devised for us. It is good to keep ourselves healthy and strong, to keep our minds and bodies fit and active. But if we continue to battle foolishly against every little wrinkle and the things we cannot change, our hearts and spirits will lose and suffer much pain in the process. We need to age respectfully and graciously with dignity and peace. If we lead good, intelligent and responsible lives, we can embrace what aging can still give us, which is love, wisdom and happiness. The most important things in life.

Section Ten - Modern Problems

Chapter Sixty - Modern Pollution.

The aim of this next section of the book is to make us a little bit more aware of some of the unfortunate things we are up against in our modern world. To try and encourage our minds to think and question more, rather than being led blindly by those whose interests in us, is not regarding our welfare but more about how they can use, manipulate, steal and profit from us. We will review several aspects of modern life and society, some of which seem intimidating and perhaps a little frightening. But don't worry, when the body and mind become strong internally, then they are more than capable of dealing with these modern threats.

Physical Pollution Of Food And Our Environment.

Mercury.

Mercury is a highly reactive toxic substance, which when ingested by the human body can lead to damage in the central nervous system, endocrine system, the kidneys and many other organs. Exposure to too much over a period of time can express itself in brain damage and ultimately death.

The mad hatter from Lewis Carroll's Alice In Wonderland is believed to have been based around mercury poisoning. As in Lewis's time in England, hatters were exposed to mercury vapours during the process of making some styles of hats. This led to many of them ending up with anxiety, confused speech and mental disorders.

These days we are predominately exposed to mercury through our consumption of fish. Although it can also be found in other animals and plant products. It has mainly come from the emissions from smoke stacks and industrial factories, which end up falling with rain on our land, sea and rivers. Coal fired powered plants are seen as the heaviest producers.

In 2009, a US geological survey tested fish from nearly 300 streams across America. This federal study found that every fish they had caught, more than a thousand altogether, had traces of mercury contamination in them. About 25 percent of these had levels higher than those the US Environmental Protection Agency considers safe for people eating average amounts of fish.

Traditionally fish, particularly those with high levels of omega oils, have been seen as a good healthy food. If levels of mercury stay as they are and do not increase in the future, then according to current government guidelines it is safe to eat up to four fish meals a week. However, for pregnant women or nursing mothers, it is recommended that they have no more than about two pieces per week. As foetuses and young children are most susceptible to harm from mercury. According to the Centres Of Disease Control in the US, about 8 percent of women of childbearing age, have enough mercury in their blood to be at risk of giving birth to children who will have subtle learning difficulties.

Fish considered to have particularly high levels of mercury are shark, sword fish, king mackerel and tile fish. Among the list of those with lower levels are shrimp, salmon, pollock, catfish, cod, haddock, sardines and trout.

Genetically Modified Foods.

With the introduction of genetically modified plants into our environment and the soon to be approved GM animal products, it seems that the human population and the entire natural world, have been turned into a massive laboratory experiment. Governments and some politicians have given into big corporations, allowing foods, which at best haven't been through enough rigorous and most importantly long term testing, to be approved and sold to us.

In the US, GM foods have been pushed on to the American public, whereas in Europe the science regarding the benefit and safety of these foods has failed to convince the European Food Agency, who have in effect banned their sale throughout Europe.

One study commissioned by the Austrian government, found that mice when fed maize as a portion of their diet, produced less and less offspring in future generations. They found that by the third and fourth litters of mice, they were producing less young and those mice still being born where now smaller in size. If this were reproduced in the public domain, it could obviously lead to catastrophic consequences for the future of the human race.

Clones.

After only six years of study, the FDA have ruled that products from cloned cattle, pigs and goats are now safe for consumers. Again the long term effects and safety of eating these animals and drinking their milk is quite unclear.

Most studies from GM and cloned foods are not coming from independent and impartial scientists, but are trials coming from those working for food companies who very clearly have their own vested interests. With cloned animals it has been found that the process produces high proportions of deformed animals. Apart from the inhumanity of this, it is certainly not very reassuring that these animals are safe to eat.

Who really knows ? Possibly they could be safe to consume. However, at the end of the day, is it really acceptable that our governments allow big business to force the public into this giant experiment.

The Food Industry.

A study in the UK in 2008 by the Children's Food Campaign, found that many major food corporations had together spent 300 million pounds per year on creating school information packs that amounted to little more than advertisements, which at times were filled with misinformation. For example, one bread making company had worksheets for children on its website which advised them to eat fruit and vegetables in moderation. Another association sponsored by leading snack and crisp manufacturers produced information for impressionable children, claiming that a bag of crisps is healthier than an apple. And yet another suggested children not reduce food intake in order to lose weight.

Nano Technology.

This involves the manipulation of molecules to make new materials. Nano particles, created from this process are ultra tiny fragments with diameters of less than 100 nanometres. A nanometre is the equivalent of one millionth of a millimetre. They are used in many products, from silver particles placed in socks to keep your feet cool and less sweaty, to being in cosmetic creams and sun tan lotion, to make them less visible and easier to apply. It is estimated that as of 2010, there are somewhere between 300 to 600 products on the marketplace using this new technology.

The concerns that are raised here come from the fact that companies have been allowed to put these products out for our use without the necessary studies required to prove their long term safety. Currently there are no government regulations in place to protect the consumer. And alarmingly independent scientists who have started to study nano particles in products like sunscreen and some diesel fuels, have found serious issues which could possibly endanger our health. They have found evidence that these ultra fine particles have moved from the skin and lungs of animals, to all the way through their systems with some particles eventually lodging in their brains. Because they are so small, once they have gathered there, the brain does not seem to have any efficient mechanism to remove them. There is speculation that in human beings these particles could play a part in neurodegenerative diseases such as Alzheimer's and Parkinson's.

Air Pollution.

A study by scientists at the University Of Washington, reported in the New England Journal Of Medicine, found that as levels of airborne pollution increased around US cities, so too did the risk of heart disease. The study reviewed 66,000 women between the ages of 50 and 79, from the Women's Health Initiative Study. It showed that for every 10 microgram rise in air pollution, this was matched by a 76 percent rise in the chances of dying from heart disease or stroke.

Another study appearing in the New England Journal Of Medicine, looked at 450,000 people over an eighteen year period. It concluded that those living in cities and exposed to the most ground level ozone pollution from car exhaust fumes and so forth, were 30 percent more likely to die from respiratory problems than those living in urban areas with the least pollution.

Water.

In 2009, the US Centres For Disease Control issued a report stating that they had found Perchlorate, a chemical used in explosives, fireworks, flares and rocket motors in 15 brands of baby milk, including the two leading brands, which accounted for 90 percent of the entire US market. Perchlorate is a potent thyroid toxin that may interfere with foetal and infant brain development. This pollution is said to mainly have come from the result of military and aerospace activities, such as the testing of rockets and missiles. Furthermore, testing has found its presence at levels considered high enough to cause problems for the unborn in public water supplies in over 35 US states.

So what else is in our water supplies? Well how about pharmaceuticals. Cancer drugs, sedatives, antibiotics, hormone replacement treatments, birth control pills, cholesterol drugs, antidepressants, and many others are now ending up in our sources of drinking water. At this stage, they are believed to be in such minute doses that they would most likely be harmless to the human being. However, the long term effects of constantly consuming traces of drugs and of combining many different types are as yet unclear and unknown.

Particularly of note is their reaction on foetuses forming in the womb and also the fertility of men, who are ingesting oestrogen like substances such as HRT and The Pill. A study part funded by the UK Environment Agency, found that male fish exposed to anti-androgen chemicals in areas near sewage outlets had female traits, such as egg cells in their testes.

These drugs are getting into our supplies through human excreta, through flushing unused drugs down the toilet and through manure from animals who have routinely ingested hormones, antibiotics and veterinary medicines, which can end up washing down into ground water. Sewage treatment facilities have not been designed to filter these drugs, so they pass fully intact through them. Along with these drugs, other chemicals are beginning to show up in our waterways, such as active ingredients and preservatives from cosmetics, detergents, toiletries and fragrances. Even trace amounts of cocaine and heroin have been found in our water.

Chemicals.

We have become surrounded by chemicals in our modern world. They are simply everywhere. It is estimated that over the last 50 years, more than 70,000 chemicals have been introduced in products around the globe. They can be found in industrial processes, cosmetics, cleaning agents, foods, plastics, paints, furniture and man made materials. Many of these chemicals have been linked to cancers, birth defects, neurological and other diseases. Some have been banned, others have not. Unfortunately it seems only after people have become sick and the damage is already done, that governments start to take action and protect the citizens who elected them.

An example of one such chemical still in use and causing recent concern, is Bisphenol A. BPA gives the clear, pliable strength to items such as plastic water bottles. It has been shown to interfere with reproductive development in animals and has been linked with infertility problems, cardiovascular disease and diabetes in humans. Research conducted at Harvard School Of Public Health found that volunteers drinking from Polycarbonate bottles, over a span of just one week, increased levels of BPA in their urine by more than two thirds, as reported in Environmental Health Perspectives. BPA can also be found in the plastic lining of some food and beverage cans.

Other chemicals such as Phthalates found in vinyl flooring, plastics, soaps, pvc and even some toothpastes, are also believed to be interfering with male hormones by mimicking properties of the female hormone oestrogen. This may be partially to blame for lower sperm counts in men, which have fallen considerably in the last 80 years. And also higher rates of testicular cancer and genital deformities in male babies.

Yet another family of chemicals, Perfluorinated chemicals, have also been linked to fertility problems and to organ damage in animals. A study by scientists at the University Of California appearing in the journal Human Reproduction found that women with the highest levels of these type of chemicals in their blood, were significantly more likely to take longer to become pregnant than those with low levels in them.

These chemicals are just the tip of the iceberg of those that surround us. Other examples include potentially toxic chemicals which have been found in some air fresheners, fragrances and laundry products.

When a scientific team at Rutgers University used common skin moisturisers in an experiment they were conducting, it was discovered by accident that these moisturisers increased the production of skin tumours by an average of 69 percent in mice who had been exposed to ultra violet light.

DEET, a chemical used in some insect repellents, which are estimated to be used by more than 200 million people worldwide each year, has been linked to damage to the nervous system and to fits in children.

The list goes on and on. At this stage in the worlds development, it seems impossible to avoid at least some exposure to external pollutants and toxins. The only good news is that if we keep our bodies reasonably clean and strong on the inside, we can avoid most of these hazardous materials from accumulating in them. The body is intelligent and will naturally try to evict anything it finds present that should not be there, be it bacteria, virus, toxin or chemical. We can hinder this process by filling up on fatty, greasy, gluey, sugary substances, which will bind and hold these unwanted chemicals into our systems, or we can help ourselves by drinking and eating bitter foods and fluid like green tea, pomegranate, berries, pineapple and grapes. These will help our bodies to flush out toxins.

We can also add in peppermint and small amounts of garlic and turmeric, which will strengthen our circulation. When combined with moderate exercise, the extra force being pushed through our blood vessels will help to dislodge any unwanted elements, allowing them to be broken up and moved to areas where they can be ejected from us.

General energy strengthening foods and exercises like deep breathing, Qigong and Yoga will also provide power for our own immune system to deal with unwanted particles in us.

On top of this we should obviously try to buy organic pesticide free foods as often as we can. We should filter our tap water and try to buy more natural products to use as cosmetics and toiletries. We can replace many chemical cleaners with natural elements such as vinegar, baking soda, lemon juice and even substances like olive oil as furniture polish. These days it is not hard to find viable and convenient easy to make alternatives, through a quick search on the internet.

It is very important to keep ourselves educated and up to date to what is going on in our world and in particular to start becoming aware that our governments who should be protecting us, are quite often failing to do so. Instead many in them are lobbied by big businesses to ignore the health and safety of consumers in order to protect their profits and vested interests.

Always give your opinions to your local elected politician and to those canvassing for votes at elections. If you feel like many others do, that it doesn't matter who gets into government, that they all behave the same way once they are there, then you should consider voting for independent candidates. If enough people use their votes this way, then the big parties will start to lose seats and on fear of losing their monopolies will be influenced to change their ways. And we will once again return to a true democratic system where the peoples voices are really being heard.

With big business, if we use our buying power to switch away from chemical laden products and choose more natural and organic ones, then they too will eventually begin to lose sales, making it economically sensible for them to switch over to produce more healthy and environmentally friendly products.

Chapter Sixty One - Social Pollution.

It is not enough that in our modern world we have to contend with all sorts of new physical threats from airborne chemicals and the contamination of our food and water, but also we now have far more mental and emotional pressures to deal with than ever before.

From a young age we are indoctrinated into a culture of consumerism, competition and manipulation, by those who have their own interests in keeping society in a certain status quo. The rich seem to be getting richer, off the hard work of many ordinary people. According to a report by the European based OECD, the income of the richest 10 percent of people in 24 developed nations was on average, nearly nine times that of the poorest 10 percent. When we continue to live in and create policies to protect a society with such inequalities, then we will continue to breed discontent and sadness in the human mind.

Through our society we have developed many of the wrong values. Values that can turn from disharmony in our minds and social lives to real physical diseases that can lower our standard of living and lead to a premature demise.

One such set of ideas surrounds work. We seem to have been taught that the idea of why we are here is not to experience, enjoy and have meaningful lives, but instead to work a minimum of eight hour days, five days a week. We seem to have allowed ourselves to become slaves in this modern era. Our governments are quite content to work not for the people and their health and happiness, but for the betterment and interests of businesses. They have now even allowed businesses to start to develop their own university degree courses, which will inevitably end up tying people to a lifetime of work for companies and corporations. We have many firms all offering up their own style diploma courses. We even have universities joining up with companies to offer tailor made degree courses for them. One such example is an English University which has joined forces with a bed manufacturing company to produce a degree in the management of selling beds.

We must not allow our education system to move any further along this path. Education should be about creating intelligent and wise minds, who will strive for innovative ways to better all our lives and not merely for the attainment of more profits on the account books of corporations.

There have been countless studies on the consequences of over work. Obviously from a Chinese perspective, it attacks and uses up energy, nutrients and hormones from the body. Leading it to a general vulnerability and weakness, which can cause illness in the mind, spirit and body on many fronts. In the West, overwork has been linked to a vast array of illnesses, such as stress, anxiety, impotence, reduced libido, depression, aggressive behaviour, addictions, insomnia, heart disease, cancer, ulcers, irritable bowel syndrome, exhaustion, burn out, chronic fatigue, and even dementia in old age.

The Finnish Institute Of Occupational Health monitored 2,214 British workers, they found that when participants in their fifties were put through a series of brain function tests, those working the longest hours scored lowest in two key tests, which were reasoning and vocabulary. The researchers felt this could lead to dementia in later life, as published in the American Journal Of Epidemiology.

A study appearing in Occupational And Environmental Health by the Karolinska Institute and Stockholm University found a strong link between stress from poor management in the work place and increased risk of episodes of heart disease, angina and heart attacks. Staff who believed their bosses to be the least competent, had a 25 percent increase in risk of heart problems. If they worked for them for four or more years, this risk increased to 64 percent.

A study by a team at the University College London appearing in the European Heart Journal, found that of the 10,000 participants, those under the age of 50 who reported that their work was stressful had 70 percent higher chance of heart disease than those who claimed their work was stress free.

So after giving the best of yourself to your job, it seems you have a far higher risk of suffering a serious, life threatening illness or one that at the very least, will lower your standards of living and your levels of happiness. The solution becomes obvious, if you are stressed at work, then change your job. Find something else that you want to do, pick something worthwhile and fulfilling that will bring meaning and value to your heart and soul. Now I know, this is very easy to say and yet can be very hard to achieve. You may initially incur lower income and other problems, but like everything else in this book, you don't have to make immediate changes, you can instead slowly start to work up to them. You can use your spare time to start to think deeply and reinterpret what really is important to you in your life, what will really bring satisfaction, reward and meaning to your existence. And then over time, you can think of ways to accomplish this. You don't have to give up your job today or tomorrow, or at all if you don't want to. But if you keep thinking in your spare time, then you should find solutions come to you, and you can find a way to make things better over the next year or two. What is most important is that you begin to take control over your life and your happiness.

Perhaps the solution with work could be convincing your employer to allow you to work a four or even three day week. This will at least give you more precious and valuable time to start living and enjoying your life. Remember we don't live in order to work, we work in order to pay for and enjoy our lives. Once you have the basics covered, somewhere to live, food on the table, heating and clothes, then get on with the living part and enjoy your life.

Chapter Sixty Two   -   The Medical Industry.

Modern Western Medicine has become somewhat sick. It has been partially compromised by big business and greed. The aim for some of those involved, is no longer Hippocrates dream of the good health and welfare of human kind, but the desire for greater and greater personal and commercial profits. In 2007, the US alone spent 2.2 trillion dollars on healthcare. A little over 250 billion of that was spent on prescription drugs.

In England, the National Health Service, has grown from having just over 93,000 nurses in 1950 to over 510,000 in 2008. From having about 8,000 doctors to nearly 40,000 over the same period of time. It has become one of the biggest employers in the world, with well over a million people working in it. Now that is a big business. One would have imagined that when numbers increased so significantly, we would now all be super healthy. But as we are aware incidents of illness are increasing and we seem to be becoming sicker and sicker. If more money was spent on education and prevention rather than on disease treatment and care, then we might find ourselves living in a very different and more healthy world.

If you were to be very cynical, you might imagine that when there is such wealth to be made from peoples illnesses, a small minority may start to take advantage of this. They might even start to believe that it makes better business sense to keep people ill and to keep them needing your treatments and drugs, rather than providing a cure and teaching them how to heal and keep themselves healthy. This type of behaviour can only be seen as very unethical, to try to make large profits from peoples suffering and misfortune.

In 2009, a study published in the New England Journal Of Medicine, found that over 5 billion US dollars had been invested, by health and life insurance businesses, into companies whose affiliates produce cigarettes, cigars and tobacco. Tobacco is considered to be the leading cause of lung cancer, and also a major factor in heart, lung and other diseases. The studies lead author, Dr. Boyd of Harvard Medical School, commented "it's clear their top priority is making money, not safeguarding peoples wellbeing".

Dangerous Or Life Enhancing New Technology ?

Gene Testing.

As technology advances other problems are starting to emerge. Gene testing is one such case. There are many companies pushing to sell gene mapping to the general public these days. They claim it can predict your future health. But as we have seen, just because you may have certain genetic markers it does not mean you will definitely get a related illness. Therefore many people who have had their genes mapped and have found negative markers, might find themselves with unnecessary stress and worry for the rest of their lives. As we will see later, stress and worry aren't just unpleasant emotions but are actually strong causes of serious diseases. So this aspect of these tests and their results may produce real harm that would not have come about otherwise.

Another aspect is if someone is told the opposite, that perhaps they have genes with low risks of heart disease or cancer for example. This could lead the person into a false sense of security which encourages them to make damaging dietary or other lifestyle choices. As genes can be switched on and off by background factors from our environment and lifestyles, then this could still lead to them becoming sick regardless as to whether they started with low risk genes or not.

CT Scans.

Another example of dangerous new technology comes in the form of Computer Tomography scans, (CT or CAT). These may be used for a multitude of different investigations. Everything from detecting kidney stones, to other problems like head trauma, internal injuries and cancer. The problem is they use large amounts of radiation to do this. A CT scan can put from 350 to 600 times the amount of radiation that an ordinary x-ray would have put into a patient. This is comparable to the amount that some of the survivors of the atomic bombs dropped on Hiroshima and Nagasaki received.

A study by scientists at Columbia University, published in the journal Radiation found that if a 45 year old has one scan, their lifetime risk of developing a cancer from it, would be about 1 in 1,200. However, quite alarmingly, if they had one scan every year for 30 years, their risk would rise to 1 in 50.

Other studies have highlighted that the risk may be even greater for children, as when they are developing, their cells are at a higher risk as they divide more rapidly, making their DNA much more vulnerable to damage from radiation.

A study published in the New England Journal Of Medicine, by a team at Columbia University

Medical Centre estimated that as much as one third of all CT scans given in the US are completely unnecessary.

Sometimes the benefits of CT scans may genuinely outweigh the risks of radiation exposure. But it is always advisable to thoroughly discuss this with your doctor and also see if other scans which do not use radiation, such as MRI, may produce as efficient results in your case.

Inventing Illnesses.

Certain companies are striving to encourage gene mapping at birth. One of the ideas behind this, is to put healthy children on drugs to prevent them getting an illness that their genes shows a risk of. However as we now know, if they have a healthy lifestyle, this alone could prevent those genes from being activated in most cases. What is also known is that many pharmaceutical medications produce side effects. This could lead to new illnesses and problems in those children who would never have gotten them otherwise.

Through clever and manipulative marketing, medicinal drugs are now being aimed at the general population. Seven academics writing a paper in the journal Nature, inferred that ordinary people, from factory workers to surgeons, would be able to boost their brain power, improve their memory and attention in the workplace, by taking stimulant drugs such as Ritalin.

This paper was quickly picked up by the media and then spread throughout the news, giving much publicity to this dangerous idea. If regulatory authorities had allowed these drugs to be marketed and sold for this purpose, it would have obviously created great financial gains for the drug makers involved. There have also been many stories spread through the media relating to the use of these drugs as aids for students in schools and universities, who could use them to enhance their abilities to learn and study for exams.

However, leaving the ethics of this aside, the other big problem with this idea is the many and increasing number of side effects now relating to these powerful stimulants. They are commonly used for the treatment of illnesses such as Attention Deficit Hyperactivity Disorder. Experts believe they act similarly to tiny doses of speed and cocaine, which sharpen the mind, allowing it to become more focused and alert.

Unfortunately, they have been linked to over fifty deaths in the US since 1999. The side effects of these type of drugs include heart problems, including heart attacks, agitation, insomnia, loss of appetite, headaches, sudden death, blood pressure, mania, stunted growth, seizures, behavioural problems, hallucinations, nervousness and vision problems. The UK's National Institute For Health And Clinical Excellence now recommends that these drugs are no longer prescribed to children under five years old, and used only for severe ADHD. Their studies found that better education and training programmes for these children and also parental training and management skills were much more productive and beneficial in the treatment of these kids.

Pharmaceutical Drugs.

In 2003, a senior executive and expert in genetics from what was then Europe's largest drug maker, gave us a startling insight into the effectiveness of pharmaceuticals. He was quoted as saying that more than 90 percent of drugs only work in 30 to 50 percent of people. He hoped that new developments in genetics would help to tailor drugs to work more specifically to increase their level of effectiveness.

Apart from the stated side effects that drug makers have found in their products. Further problems can arise when drugs are mixed with other drugs. This can lead to many interactions and is a common problem. According to US statistics, two thirds of people over 65 and three quarters of people over 80 have multiple chronic health conditions needing many medications. It has become hard to tell if many of those extra medications are being given to treat the original diseases or to treat new conditions caused by side effects of original medications.

When drug manufacturers are running trials to prove the efficacy of their new drug they often hand pick the participants, excluding anyone who may make their drug look ineffective or may have higher chances of side effects. Often people who have more than one illness will not be allowed into trials, as they are more difficult and complex to treat successfully. It is estimated that over 80 percent of trials exclude these types of people. The problem is that if the new drug is approved then these are the very types of patients who will be using it. And therefore the effects and side effects in them will be less than clear.

An example of drugs working in theory in comparison to the real world, was recently provided by a study from the Imperial College London. They studied over 4000 people in twelve European countries, who were taking medications for cardiovascular disease. They found that only one in four people in the study on blood pressure drugs reached their target level, one in three on cholesterol drugs reduced it to the required level and about one in two had success in managing their diabetes with medications.

Bad Medical Decisions.

Another problem with drugs and even tests and surgical procedures is the influence of money. We have an odd and naive belief that everyone involved in medicine is honest and will always give you a truthful opinion. That they will not exaggerate the benefits of a procedure or a drug and will also clearly highlight any side effects or risks that may be associated with it. But just like with every other business there are always good and bad people to be found. So it is highly likely that there will be some who put their wealth before their patients well being, they may suggest patients take drugs that may be no good for them, or even put themselves through surgery which could be dangerous and yet be of no benefit.

Because of the often very large sums of money involved, you may also find that subconsciously some doctors and scientists may perhaps exaggerate test and study results rather than giving completely unbiased assessments. These problems could be easily resolved if governments were to create more impartial guidelines for the medical industry. Such as having one set of doctors to diagnose surgical conditions and another unrelated set to perform the surgeries. In that way you could be guaranteed that money has not consciously or subconsciously influenced your surgeons decision to perform an operation.

Even bullying and intimidation by patients can cause ordinary doctors to make poor decisions. Such is the case with commonly prescribed antibiotics. It was believed at one stage that these drugs were useful in treating disorders like the common cold, flu and sore throats. So now when patients go to a clinic with one of those conditions, some often demand antibiotics. Many doctors under this pressure will hand them out. But they are aware that antibiotics will not be helpful in curing these viral conditions and may even be dangerous. According to the US Centre For Disease Control, clinical trials quite clearly demonstrate that antibiotics are only effective for bacterial infections. Their own study published in Clinical Infections Diseases found that antibiotics were responsible for about 142,000 emergency departments visits in the US every year. Ranging from rashes to allergies to anaphylaxis, which can be life threatening.

There are numerous drugs and procedures that have been used in Western Medicine which have shown themselves to be at best ineffective and at worst to be damaging or even deadly.

An example is Vertebroplasty, where doctors inject a type of cement into fractured back bones. It is performed about 40,000 times a year in the US. When two separate studies reported in the New England Journal Of Medicine compared it to fake or placebo treatment, they both found no difference in patients up to six months later who had real surgery compared to fake treatment.

Two other trials for a procedure called arthroscopic knee surgery for the condition osteoarthritis of the knee, found that the treatment which had been performed about 180,000 times a year in the US, again was no better than sham placebo surgery.

Common treatments clomid and IUI for infertility problems were found in a trial by Aberdeen University, reported in the British Medical Journal, to have no real benefits in increasing pregnancies. Another fertility procedure using frozen eggs has only about a 6 percent chance of success according to the British Fertility Society. Yet some clinics have led women to believe they can safely have their eggs frozen as they pursue a career or wait for their ideal partner to show up.

A study by McMasters University appearing in the Lancet discovered that beta blockers used to reduce blood pressure before heart surgery, actually found that patients who took them prior to surgery were one third more likely to die within a month than those given a fake pill. It was also found to increase the incidents of strokes.

A study by Copenhagen University, appearing in the journal Gastroenterology, discovered that when healthy participants took proton pump inhibitors for eight weeks, many of them actually ended up developing the symptoms of heartburn and indigestion, the very same symptoms these drugs are designed to treat. These drugs are among the biggest selling in the world, with an estimated 5 percent of the developed worlds' population using them. They have also strongly been linked to the brittle bone disease osteoporosis. One study by at team at he University of Manitoba in Canada, reported in the Canadian Medical Association Journal, that after using them regularly for five years, there was a 44 percent higher risk of hip fracture. After seven years this rose to 400 percent.

A review of 47 clinical trials by the University Of Hull, published in the Journal Plos Medicine, found that common anti-depressants had hardly any clinical effect on depressed patients. They found they had a relatively small effect on people with severe depression but had no more effect than a dummy pill on people with mild or moderate depression. The difference with this study was the fact that the researchers, using the Freedom Of Information laws, were able to gain access to previously unpublished and withheld drug trial data. And with this new information a clearer, less favourable picture of the anti-depressants efficacy emerged.

Chapter Sixty Three - Prevention Versus Treatment.

The vast majority of money spent in Western Medicine is not on health care but on disease care. Money is spent on creating new drugs and new technologies and treatments, rather than on education and prevention. People are lulled into a false sense of security by dreams of magic pills and futuristic machines and computer chips, which will manage and enhance their bodies without any effort from them. This leads them to believe that they can make reckless decisions in their lives without any serious consequences or negative comebacks.

However, the truth is that it is far easier to remain in good condition and disease free by following a reasonably healthy diet and lifestyle, than it is to enter the medical system, where drugs and procedures are used to try and patch the body up after the damage is done. And if you do enter it without making any change, you will most likely find, the problems remain and new ones quite often start to appear as well.

Unless the real root of the problem is addressed, drugs if effective, very often do not cure the issue and make you healthy, but may instead just suppress and mask it. By creating the symptoms in the first place, the body is often trying to warn us and tell us that we are on the wrong path in life, and we must change our ways. Taking a pill or having surgery is at best a quick fix, leaving us still to make the deeper real lifestyle changes that are required if we want our good health to return.

For example, taking anti-psychotic drugs or anti-depressants without dealing with the mental, emotional or other issues that caused the illness is obviously not a long term solution.

With cancer, although chemotherapy, radiotherapy and surgery may be effective in some cases. They do not address why the cancer appeared in the first place, nor prevent the chances of it returning again years later to perhaps a different part of the body.

Bypass surgeries and stents are only effective in dealing with an emergency cardiovascular situation. The patient needs to change their diet and life to really successfully treat and remove all the sludge and fats that has built up in their arteries. And also to deal with issues of stress that may be straining their heart, if they seriously want to have any real chance of reducing their risk of another major heart event.

Other well known illnesses like Type II Diabetes can be prevented through the consumption of a healthy diet. In many cases, it can even be effectively treated if a patient changes their diet and rids bad fats and sugars from it. Diet is clearly the biggest factor involved in Type II Diabetes. In the last twenty years, the Chinese have gone from eating a good natural diet and having very low levels of this illness, to eating a diet rich in Western style foods and sugars, and now having nearly as high levels of this disease as found in the US.

Another example of treatment versus prevention can be seen in cholesterol lowering statins. These drugs help to remove bad fats from your blood, but in the process they also seem to remove the good oils too. As negative side effects seem to be mounting for these drugs, many are beginning to question their widespread use. Side effects of low levels of good oils and good cholesterol include memory problems, reduced intelligence, depression, aggression and violent acts, anxiety, muscle pain and damage, gastro-intestinal problems, headaches, joint pains, nerve damage, sleep disturbance, sexual dysfunctions, and suicide. Whereas by simply having a healthy diet your body will naturally have low levels of bad cholesterol and high levels of the good one, making you feel good and reduce your risks of many diseases as well. It is also worth noting, that if you take statins and still continue to have a bad diet, you may end up with low cholesterol but still high risks of many other problems.

Today we are taking more and more drugs than ever, we are having more procedures and have developed a huge industry around illness. We are spending trillions on disease care every year. We have done everything but actually tackle the real culprits behind illness. And until we start to wake up and see there is a limit to the effectiveness of Western Medicine in its current form of trying to patch up the body after it has become sick, and then start to take responsibility for our own bodies and their well being, we will unfortunately be caught in this vicious circle of symptoms, drugs, procedures and then even more symptoms. Personal responsibility with good diet and lifestyle are the only true ways to attain health in the body, mind and spirit.

It is also becoming a dangerous thing to be sick these days, not just from the illness itself, but from the treatment of it. Nearly every time you take a Western medical drug or enter a hospital to have some form of surgery, you are exposing yourself to a possible chance of side effects, errors and complications. Everything from adverse drug reactions, to surgical complications, to hospital acquired infections. From evidence given to the UK governments House Of Commons Health Committee in 2008, it is estimated that up to 40,000 people die in the UK every year from problems created by the Western medical system. The committee was informed that the most reliable evidence suggested, 10 percent of all patients admitted to hospitals suffered harm from their treatment.

It is believed by most experts that side effects and errors are vastly under reported. There are many reasons for this. For starters, doctors are usually too busy to find time to fill out complicated reports on incidents. Then there is the question of liability, a health care worker may be reluctant to take responsibility for an incident which may damage their careers, and also because of our culture of claims and compensations, burden their financial incomes. Even personal pride can have an impact. No one really wishes to own up to things and admit they have made errors.

As this subject is a part of Western Medicine that is unglamorous and highlights its weaknesses, there have been very few studies in this area. One such study was carried out by Dr. Starfield, a professor of public health at the famous John Hopkins Hospital. Her study analysed the number of deaths from medical treatment in the US, using data gathered between 1993 and 1998. It was published in the prestigious Journal Of The American Medical Association. Her report found the following, 12,000 deaths from unnecessary surgery, 7,000 deaths from medication errors in hospitals, 20,000 deaths from other errors in hospitals, 80,000 deaths from infections acquired in hospitals and 106,000 deaths from non-error adverse effects of medications. In total, these amounted to an estimated 225,000 deaths each year from medical causes, which would make

Western Medicine the third leading cause of death in the US, after heart disease and cancer. Since then, other studies have indicated that this figure may be considerably higher in the US.

Having read all that, please be aware that the purpose of this chapter is not to frighten us away from getting medical treatment, it is just to highlight that it is not risk free and that the more responsibility you take on board for yourself, the safer and healthier you can be. Obviously if you are sick, you cannot just ignore it, and need to get some form of proper treatment, be it Chinese, Western or some other form of medicine.

If you are receiving healthcare, there are many steps you can take to reduce any associated errors and complications from it. You can start by making sure you ask lots of questions about your illness and its proposed treatment. It is better to make a written list of these questions rather than trying to rely on your memory, particularly as you may become nervous or stressed in the consultation. The internet can provide invaluable information on most illnesses, surgeries and related drugs used for them. It is not hard from there to devise lots of good questions for your physician.

Do also remember that it is your body and your right to ask for lots of information, Western Medicine is now more than ever a business, and drugs, surgeries and other treatments are products in it. People working in this industry are highly compensated. Although many of these people have good intentions, the bottom line is that it is not a charity, but a business which is after profit, just the same as any other business. So like every other service, thoroughly examine what you are being offered before getting deeply involved in it.

If you are prescribed prescription drugs, be sure to enquire how effective they are, and ask lots of question such as, will they just suppress symptoms or will they treat the underlying condition, are there any other alternatives to using them, are there changes you can make to your lifestyle and diet instead of taking them, and is there a plan to get you back off the medication.

When taking drugs be sure to read the accompanying leaflet for any adverse side effects. Also a quick search on the internet can make you aware if other patients taking the same drug have had any complications from it. If you do start to experience any known side effects or any other new problems, obviously be sure to return your doctor as soon as possible. Always ask them to report these side effects back to the manufacturer, as this may help to make the system safer in the future.

If you are going for surgery, be sure to ask about success and risk rates involved in the operation. Don't just presume that if an operation is carried out that it has high success rates or is safe and without risk. Do your own investigative research, and if you become uncertain then it is advisable to get a second opinion from an independent source. It is also worthwhile bringing a friend or relative with you to consultations. They can take notes for you and also ask questions you may have forgotten.

As occasional mistakes can be made through poor communications between doctors, nurses, technicians and hospital departments, it is a good idea to keep extra personal copies of all your reports, test results and prescriptions. Although most doctors and nurses usually do a good job, you may be unfortunate to be the unlucky one who comes across a doctor, who due to being too stressed, too busy or some other reason, makes a mistake. The best way to avoid this is to get to know all about your treatments, medications and correct dosages. Then you can simply interact with the medical team treating you and remind them if they have seemed to forgotten something relevant.

Most doctors, scientists and health care workers are good people. Many of them started off with sincere intentions to help others, but as the medical industry has gotten bigger and bigger, they too have become a casualty. They no longer have time to spend with their patients and now often rely on test results, rather than the old style of face to face communication and examinations. They no longer have the time to get to know the more human side of their patients. This has led many of them to feel less rewarded by their work, and instead to feel more pressured and stressed.

Many are now dragged along by the system and have no alternative but to give out some drugs that they might not have full confidence in. Such was the case with the recent Swine Flu vaccines. Where a poll of doctors taken in England for Pulse magazine showed that 49 percent of doctors would refuse the vaccine for personal use, on the grounds that it had not been tested enough.

It is time for a rethink of parts of Western Medicine, to turn it back into Hippocrates original vision of one which will help and strengthen all of society. From both Chinese medical theories and Western medical scientific studies we now have a clear picture of how to obtain health, and the happiness that stems from it. Governments need to redirect the focus and finances of Western Medicine away from disease care and towards real prevention of illness and promotion of health.

Section Eleven   -   Emotions And The Mind

Chapter Sixty Four   -   Emotional Health.

Chinese Medicine takes a very different and much more developed approach to the mind and the emotions in comparison to the way they are treated in the West. In Western Medicine, although they often try to give you chemicals to boost the brain, depression and other mental health issues are mostly considered to come from external problems in a persons life and are treated by psychiatrists and psychologists.

However in the East, the mind, emotions, body, energy and spirit are all inseparable and every one of them can affect the others when weak or diseased.

For example, weak adrenal glands can fail to produce enough adrenalin which causes you to generally become more fearful in life. This could be caused by a physical source, such as overexposure to cold which steals the energy from the kidneys and adrenal glands, and makes them underproductive, or it may also have come from an emotional source, such as harassment and pressure in work, which over time and repeated calls on your kidneys for hormones to deal with the stress could lead them to weaken and tire out. Either way, without the affect of the adrenalin, the mind and the heart will become unsteady and you may end up being jumpy, easily rattled and more nervous.

As we will see shortly, each organ has a strong impact on the emotional activity of the brain. Emotions aren't just caused by external events, as commonly believed in Western Medicine, but can also be caused by the failure of proper functioning of each of the organs. And in turn, if strong emotions cause a reaction in the mind, the mind will not be alone in suffering but a chain of events will occur throughout the physical and energetic body. These may lead to its weakening or breakdown, producing real physical ailments, from heart disease, to cancer, to digestive problems, to skin diseases and a whole host of others. Weaknesses in energy, blood and Jing can also cause many problems for the mind and emotions. Everything is connected and cannot be neatly put away into separate categories. When one part gets sick, it can and usually does affect many others.

Chapter Sixty Five - The Influence Of The Liver And The Heart.

(It is worth noting at this point that as I discussed earlier, when we talk of organs in Chinese Medicine, it is not just their physical presence we are speaking of, but their entire sphere of influence on everything they affect in the human being. From the physical to the energetic, to the mental, emotional and spiritual).

The Liver.

The liver has a huge impact on the mood in Chinese Medicine. Particularly in terms of controlling low moods, mood swings, irritability, frustration and anger.

The Liver performs hundreds of functions. In Chinese Medicine one of the most important of these, is the regulation and smooth flow of blood and energy into the body. The Liver turns carbohydrates from your food into glucose in the blood stream. If the liver becomes unhealthy or is overworked, it may fail to release blood and the energy it contains into your system.

The body constantly needs differing amounts of blood and energy in circulation. When you are mentally active or physically busy, such as working out in a gym, the body and in this particular case the muscles will need more blood and energy. Whereas when you are resting, such as lying in bed, the body requires less blood. The Liver is in charge of managing the volume of blood in circulation in your system, it holds or releases blood when it is needed throughout the day and night.

The consequences of failing to manage this blood are very important. On the physical side, with less blood and the oils contained within, the muscles will become stiff, achy and tight, making you uncomfortable and more easily agitated. This is a similar experience to the up-tightness you feel when you get stressed. Muscles need lubricants and oils to remain supple. In nature, if we look at a tree which is healthy with plenty of oil and sap in it, its branches can be pushed and pulled but will always spring back into place. If however, the tree is dried out, its branches start to creek and strain when bent, and inevitably snap and break. When muscles are without sufficient oils and blood they too become sore and tight. And will rip and sprain more easily.

So this physical effect has already started to make you feel uncomfortable, but it doesn't end there. The lack of control of proper release of blood from the liver means that the mind will not get all that is required to keep it strong, nourished and powered up. Without sufficient blood and the nutrients, energy and hormones carried within it, the mind will start to lose its spark, just as the light from a torch starts to fade when the batteries get weak. Even vision and hearing may be affected. With colours losing their vibrancy and sounds losing their sharpness.

In Chinese Medicine, the liver can be seen as one of the culprits causing depression. The classical symptoms being irritability and mood swings. Mood swings are caused by the livers mismanagement of blood throughout the day. When more blood is requested for activity, if the liver has not enough energy to deliver it, the mood and general energy levels will drop leaving you tired and in low spirits.

Another way the liver and its partner the gallbladder can affect the mind is through the production of bile. Bitter bile breaks down fats and accumulations throughout the body and brain, if production of bile reduces, this can lead to a build up of unwelcome sludge in your system. This can block up parts of the body causing aches and pains, which tends to make you feel more agitated, but may also block up the brain causing interference with mental processing and leading to confused and irrational thoughts and indecisiveness.

The last effect the liver has on the mind can lead to one of the strongest emotions, which is anger and even to rage as it intensifies. How could it possibly do this ? Well quite simply through the medium of heat. As the liver is doing such a vast number of functions it can start to generate lots of heat, this heats the blood it is holding and also the blood passing through it. Heat causes fluids to expand and atoms and molecules to vibrate and bounce off each other. Heat also tends to rise. So all this hot swollen active blood tends to rush up into your head and starts to cause pressure in your skull. Your face gets hot. Your eyes may get blood shot. Your blood vessels may begin to throb. You become like a pressure cooker waiting to explode. To further compound this, in a stressful situation, you start to tense up, as energy tries to push through all this tightness it starts to generate even more heat in the body.

Anger is a very hot emotion and all our common expressions clearly associate it with heat and pressure. Hot headed, hot tempered, burning with rage, letting off steam, he went red with anger, veins throbbed in his forehead, he was ready to burst, his blood was boiling and so on. The opposite can be said for being relaxed. Such as, he was chilled, cool and calm. We even have the word livid, obviously derived from the word liver, which is used to describe frustration and irritability. We also have liverish, and bilious from the word bile, used to describe someone with a crabby and disagreeable disposition. Maybe our European ancestors knew a lot more about the workings of the liver and its effects on the mind, than modern medicine would have us believe.

To sum up the liver, its negative effects on the mind can be generally portrayed through low moods, mood swings, irritability, up tightness, tension, agitation, resentment, bottling up and holding emotions, stubbornness, frustration, anger, rage, and scatty and illogical decision making. When the liver is in good health, the mind is usually clear headed, in a good steady mood and the demeanour is relaxed and easy going.

Physical illnesses stemming from liver heat and pressure can be headaches, pains and aches, twitches, spasms, tight and stiff muscles, rashes and skin problems, red and dry eyes, cramps, insomnia, brittle and dry nails, strokes, cancer, heart attacks, painful periods and menstrual problems, ulcers and irritable bowel syndrome, alopecia and hair loss.

How To Help Your Liver System.

What can we do if we find ourselves with an overworked and overheated liver ? Well general good health such as prescribed in the rest of the book is very helpful and over the long term should help to bring the liver back into good health and balance.

If you have access to Chinese herbs and a herbalist, then there are some formulas such as Xiao Yao Wan, loosely referred to as free and easy wanderer pills, which are really effective and excellent in creating a good and steady mood. However as emotional conditions can be very deep in the body, you may sometimes have to take herbs for long periods before health returns and you get the required effect. You will need to consult with a Chinese Herbalist for advice on your particular circumstance, if you wish to take herbs.

Stress, frustration and anger are the emotions which will have the most damaging effect on the liver. There are a great deal of mental and spiritual methods that can be used to curtail them and counter any problems caused by them. There are many ways you can influence the mind to create a physical effect within the body, these will be discussed in the next few chapters.

Moderate exercise is also beneficial in moving liver energy and blood. Helping to both invigorate and cool it. However over exercise will often over tire the liver and damage it, so keep it moderate.

And of course there is food. If you are prone to anger and stress, avoid foods that heat and dry or form toxins in the body, such as hot spices, alcohol, coffee, dark teas, sugars, fats, red meat and dairy. To cool things down you need to add in bitter juices, fruit and green tea.

Peppermint tea is also very useful for the liver, to cool it and to help it move liver energy, blood and circulation through the body, allowing the mind and muscles to be properly fed, cooled and nourished by the extra blood supply and its ingredients. Good plant oils also help smooth movement through the body, they can ease the workload of the liver and prevent the body tightening during stressful periods.

The Heart.

The heart is a wonderful organ. It is powered up by an electrical pulse. In the space of a minute, it has pumped about eight pints of blood right the way through your body. If you live for eighty years, it will have managed to beat around three billion times without stopping to take a break or a rest.

In Chinese Medicine, such is its importance amongst the organs, that it is seen as the emperor of the body, in charge of the smooth running of your entire system. In good health it does this incredibly well, however in poor health it will quickly diminish your standard of living and even end up in many cases being the most likely cause of your demise.

Heart attacks or myocardial infarctions to give them their full Western Medical name, are responsible for more deaths than any other cause in the developed world. In the US, a man or woman is stricken by a heart attack about every 30 seconds. About every 55 seconds someone unfortunately dies from one. And yes you read that right, every other person who gets a heart attack dies from it. It is not at all like on TV medical shows and programs, where people seem to routinely and easily recover from such events.

In a recent study by a team at the University of Washington, it was discovered that patients suffering cardiac arrest, where problems with the electrical signals in the heart can cause it to stop functioning properly, had only on average a 4.6 percent chance of survival in the US if the event occurred outside of a hospital. This increased a small amount to 8.4 percent survival in those who were treated by emergency responders at the scene of the incident.

More than 80 percent of cases of cardiac arrest occur in people with coronary artery disease, were their arteries have become clogged with cholesterol and other toxins.

It becomes even more depressing when the events after a major heart incident become known. Problems like heart attacks cause damage to the muscle of the heart, which over time hardens into stiff scar tissue. This can develop into heart failure, whereby the scarring has caused the heart to become inflexible and unable to contract and pump blood efficiently. It is estimated in the US, that about 22 percent of men and 46 percent of women will develop heart failure within approximately six years of a heart attack. The diagnosis is poor, less than half the patients survive more than five years after the initial diagnosis, and only a quarter are alive after ten years.

In Chinese Medicine hearts can be damaged and weakened by foods that leave too much phlegm and fat in your blood vessels, by over exercising which can strain the heart, and by the emotions. Many emotions can have an impact on the heart but the ones that affect it the most are loneliness, sadness, over excitement and anxiety. Just like with the other organs, it goes both ways, emotions can have a physical impact on the heart and a physically weak or ill heart can impact on the functioning of the mind and the mood to produce negative emotions.

Ultimately continuous stress and damage on the heart may most likely lead it to a heart attack.

If you do manage to survive a heart attack, your life will still inevitably change for the worse, so before putting yourself through all that hardship and suffering, think about doing the easier and simpler changes now, which will not just save your future health but will also make you happier in your present state.

An Over Stimulated Heart.

Over excitement, even if coming from a supposedly good event can over stimulate and over burden the heart, causing it to heat and speed up. This can cause the mind to start to overheat and it can also interfere with levels of blood and oxygen it is receiving. Which may lead your mind to over thinking, becoming anxious and wound up, to insomnia and difficulty sleeping. You may even notice your thoughts become scattered and confused. There may be feelings of pressure or tightness in your chest. Your breathing may be shallow or erratic and your heart may suffer palpitations, irregular rhythms or flutters.

This condition will be worsened by exposure to many elements of modern life, such as a stressful, demanding, busy and pressurised job, and stimulants like coffee, alcohol, cigarettes, drugs, and strong spices. It can also be exacerbated by a hectic social and general lifestyle, chronic and long term stress and anxiety, particularly in relationships. And it may even originate from many of our modern methods of escapism, such as gripping TV programs, movies and computer games.

In this scenario the heart has often become hot, tired and over worked. Its energy has weakened. It needs time out and away from busy activities and stressful situations.

This will help it cool and re-gather its energy and power. If your heart has found itself in this state, you need to seriously think about changing to a more calm and balanced lifestyle. If you continue to put the heart under such pressure, it may age it, damage it, overwork it, exhaust it and eventually stop it and you in your tracks.

For an overheated heart you can also eat plenty of cooling mineral filled foods like vegetables and in particular beet root, seaweed, kelp and spirulina. Also avoid stimulants like coffee, alcohol and hot spices until the heat has gone.

A Weakened Heart.

The heart has the responsibility of pumping blood, energy, and oxygen into your brain at a steady and continuous rate in order for your memory and mental faculties to work sharply and precisely. If however the heart is altered, if it becomes irregular, if it perhaps loses its strength and the flow of blood through it weakens, then the blood may not pick up enough oxygen as it is passed through the lungs. In turn as it moves and is pumped more unsteadily through the mind, the mind too may get a far too limited supply of blood and what it is receiving has insufficient energy and oxygen. With less fuel, the brain will be less able to compute, perceive, understand and think logically.

Under these circumstances the mind may even find it difficult to communicate with the outside world. To compound this, when it finds itself in such a situation, it often becomes startled and panics. This unfortunately places even more demands to deliver more blood and oxygen, on an already struggling heart, and often causes it to tense under the pressure, producing even less. Socially this can leave even a very intelligent person left blank and looking like a dummy and lost for words. Persistent communication problems stemming from a weak or malfunctioning heart can leave you feeling separated, lonely and disconnected from the world and can lead to many of the established Western psychiatric disorders.

This problem is essentially caused by weak heart energy. Usually the patient will have more general feelings of cold and tiredness. Physical exhaustion and over exercise are strong culprits. Low calorie diets and lack of nutrients and nourishment, continuous pressure and long term stress, chronic illness, over exposure to cold weather, bad relationships and overwork or study can also be all factors leading to this condition.

Again taking a break and giving your heart time to recuperate and regain its energy and strength is very important. Avoid hard work, stress and intense exercise. Instead get plenty of rest and eat lots of nourishing energy and blood building foods such as white rice, raisins, mushrooms, nuts, seeds and olive oil. Also have small amounts of weak coffee, alcohol, bitter chocolate, honey and spices, in particular turmeric and garlic. Add in these stimulants in small amounts and build up their effect until they have created the right amount of energy to help power up the heart but not enough to over stimulate it.

The Heart And Loneliness.

Probably the most damaging condition for the heart is loneliness. Feeling isolated, excluded, rejected and separate from the rest of the world can seriously weaken and deplete heart energy, leading to many negative repercussions throughout the body. When the heart gets weak, everywhere gets less blood, oxygen, energy and nutrients and thus weakens and suffers. Most people have felt the effects of a broken heart when a romantic relationship ends. They don't just feel anxiety, despair and sadness in their minds but they can often feel physical tightness, pain and aching in their chest too.

We commonly associate love and loneliness with the heart in Western culture. From romantic symbols of hearts on cards for Valentines Day, to phrases like heart ache, heart was crushed and broken hearted in references to relationships that end badly.

However loneliness is not just to do with lack of romance, nor is it just purely from isolation, but it can also be found in people when they are surrounded by others. In this circumstance, it is more to do with feeling disconnected, different and not understood or accepted by others. This is a problem that has stemmed from our society, which as we were growing up, drummed into our subconscious minds that we should constantly seek the attention and approval of others even if we believe differently to them. Thanks to this bad programming, people now often feel out of place and rejected if they are not fitting in with the crowd. Advertisers and those in positions of power often use and abuse this technique in order to manipulate you into buying their products and conforming to their rules. Some of the techniques in the following chapters helps the mind to become more aware and gives it the ability needed to avoid this sort of modern day bullying.

When an individual suffers from a lack of love or connection, from loneliness over a long period of time, many physical symptoms from the heart may start to appear. Such as flutters, palpitations, irregular rhythms, fast or slow heartbeat, breathlessness, tiredness, chest pain or tightness, cold hands and feet, weakness and paleness. Furthermore the lack of good circulation will affect all the other organs, leading to problems arising in and increasing from them. The mind too will be affected and a wide range of problems may occur, such as anxiety, depression, sadness, inability to communicate, avoiding eye contact, speech problems, panic attacks, difficulty smiling, nervous smiling, unsettled or racing mind, being over self conscious, scattered and flustered mind, over excitable, easily embarrassed, poor memory, sleep problems, shyness and avoiding social contact.

Meditation, positive affirmations, Qi Gong, Shen Gong, Yoga and other mind work can all be very beneficial to healing and strengthening the heart and mind. The simple practice of unconditional love and happiness, of finding genuine meaning and spirituality, can, if guided in the right ways, work wonders for the heart and the rest of you too. We will discuss many of these methods shortly.

Chapter Sixty Six - The Influence Of The Other Major Organs.

We have already discussed the lungs, kidneys and digestive organs in previous chapters. So in this segment we will just briefly recap on them.

The Lungs.

Poor physical lung function can often create a steady drop in mood. As the two main jobs of the lungs are to take in air and to excrete waste, if they fail to effectively take in enough oxygen, your energy levels will slump and both your body and mind will lose power and become tired. An over tired mind often loses its sparkle leading to depressed thoughts and actions.

So too can the opposite occur, where the mind impacts on the lungs. If the mind becomes sad, disappointed, suffers the loss of a loved one or even loses hope, the shoulders often droop forward, the lungs slump and the back hunches over. If this is being repeated over a period of time the physical lungs may weaken and become damaged. When the lungs are constricted, oxygen cannot enter and be passed effectively around the body. Energy levels will drop, and as they do the mind and mood will lower even more so. Like many of the other emotions, a vicious circle begins, where the original cause creates a knock on effect which further creates a downward spiral.

Another emotional effect stemming from the lungs, can be a sense of feeling trapped and suffocated. When the lungs are unable to fill and empty properly, it can lead to a claustrophobic sensation which generates a feeling of fear, panic, paranoia and loss of control in the mind. If this happens at night while asleep, it can turn dreams into nightmares.

The last mental effect on the mind, to come from the lungs is more of a general one relating to toxins. As lung capacity lowers, the ability to remove toxins from the body reduces causing a build up of them in the blood stream. They will of course eventually end up in the mind. Where they can lodge and block connections leading to confusion, irrational behaviour and poor judgement. In Chinese Medicine, if toxins are left in the mind over the long term, it can lead to more permanent blockages and damages to produce senility and eventually diseases like Alzheimer's. A build up of toxins can of course come from many sources in the body and not just poor lung functioning.

To clear the lungs, small amounts of aromatic spices that move energy are useful. These will melt and expectorate phlegm from the lungs and head, allowing them to open up, breathe more effectively and pass circulation more easily to and through the brain. Peppermint will also help to cool and move Qi in the lungs and head.

If your lungs are toxic and hot, then add cooling bitter foods such as pomegranate, grape, green tea and berries into the mix. These will clean the lungs and open and loosen the bowel movement, helping toxins to be passed out of the intestine and away from the lungs, relieving the pressure on them.

Because of the deep abdominal and complete breathing involved in Qi Gong and Yoga exercises, these are often very beneficial in dealing with lung disorders and in strengthening them up. This helps to supply extra oxygen to the brain which enhances its mental functioning and stimulates positive moods.

The Digestive Organs.

If our digestion fails to break down our food properly then we will simply not have enough raw materials to build all the chemicals, such as serotonin, that our brains need to keep our moods elevated. Our energy levels may also drop, lowering the power supply to the brain and even to our eyes and ears and other senses, reducing their ability to perceive events around us in their true vibrant forms.

Another effect of a weak digestion is that it will not break down foods properly, leaving thicker, heavier, undigested particles in the blood stream, which in turn creates phlegm and mucus. This blocks up the mind causing poor memory and concentration, and confused and muddled thoughts. This can prevent you from thinking clearly and seeing solutions to your problems which leads the mind to over thinking and worry from the inability to resolve problems.

Sometimes the digestion is not weak but has become dirty and blocked up on the inside. When this happens the putrid fluids and phlegm lining the inside of the intestine may stop and prevent good nutrients from your food being absorbed into your blood stream, leading to a shortfall in the mind. And from there over the long term, this can create depression. It may also cause heat, toxins and phlegm to gather in the brain leading to anxiety, irrational thoughts, psychiatric disorders and dementia.

If our digestion has become weak and cold with symptoms such as tiredness after eating, loose bowel movements without much or any odour, clear urine, feelings of cold in the body and paleness in the face. Then add plenty of white rice to your diet and small amounts of spices and a little alcohol with meals a few times a week as well.

If it is toxic and overheated, usually the strongest symptoms will be heartburn and bad breath if the stomach is hot and dirty. And odorous gas, yellow urine and odorous bowel movements or constipation if the intestines have become so. In these cases stay clear of fats, sugars and toxins, spices and coffee, red tea and alcohol. And also add in cooling and detoxifying green tea, peppermint tea and bitter fruits and juices to clean them out.

The Kidneys.

The kidneys create the emotion of fear in the mind. If your kidneys have become weak and you do not have enough strong stimulant hormones in your blood, then most likely you will find that you have become jumpy, nervous, easily startled and fearful. Hormones like cortisol, adrenalin and testosterone make you strong, brave and fearless. If you have exhausted or run down your reserves of then you may find that situations can easily over come you, often leaving you nervous and jittery on the inside. Your will power too, will weaken. You quite simply won't have as much vigour and get up and go in your life.

Too muck work, exercise or even partying, are all things that can wear your hormones out. But also too much stress and in particular shocks and frights, can quickly deplete your hormones.

When your body receives a bad shock, one where you have not been physically touched, where the whole incident came through your senses, mind and perception. Then if you are low on hormones, you can easily see how quickly bodily effects can come about from an effect not perpetrated on your physical person but solely on your mind. You could pass out, vomit, wet yourself or defecate, your knees could go from under you, your heart start to race in your chest, you could start to lose your vision or hearing, you could tremble or break out into a cold sweat and so on. With a shock it is often very quick and dramatic to see the instantaneous physical effects of mental emotions.

To strengthen hormones and kidney energy, avoid doing too much, be it work, partying, exercise or anything else. Eat lots of nourishing foods like walnuts and pumpkin seeds, eggs, oils, mushrooms, and add in a touch of salt and cinnamon to astringe and hold the hormones in your body.

As Qi Gong and Yoga will generate lots of extra and spare energy in your system, they are both very useful in relieving the workload and any pressure on the kidneys to release hormones to boost up the body. The kidneys and adrenal glands will therefore get a well deserved rest, allowing them to recuperate, preserve your Jing and strengthen themselves back up. So Yoga, and Qi Gong in particular, are highly recommended for healing your kidneys and preserving your Jing.

Chapter Sixty Seven   -   Negative Emotions Throughout Life.

Obviously at any stage in your life, you can pass through a difficult time and find yourself being affected by negative emotions and their physical reactions in the body. However, many people suffer the most damage early on in their lives. We have already seen in an earlier chapter how someone may not only be affected by inheriting emotional patterns of behaviour from their parents, but also even stress placed upon the mother during pregnancy can have a long lasting negative effect on the child.

As the child grows, stress, bullying and neglect may come from many areas in their lives. In the past it came from parents, teachers, other kids at school and so forth. Nowadays, we can throw many TV programs and presenters, commercials and advertising onto that list. All more than willing to prey on vulnerable young minds to push sales, egos and agendas.

In a report for the Children's Society in England it was claimed, that the aggressive pursuit of personal success by adults is now the greatest threat to children. Many parents are now putting their own quests for pleasure before that of their kids, which will inevitably lead to higher incidence of mental and emotional problems for all concerned in the future. The same report cited research claiming that three year olds who lived with lone parents were three times as likely to have behavioural problems as those who lived with married parents. It also suggested that children with separated parents were 50 percent more likely to fail at school, have self esteem issues, be unpopular and have behavioural difficulties, anxiety or depression.

A study examining responses to a psychological questionnaire, The Minnesota Multiphasic Personality Inventory, from over 77,0000 US students between 1938 and 2007, discovered that five times as many students were now dealing with anxiety than the number who suffered from it during the era of the great depression when the questionnaire began. One area in particular, hypomania, increased over six fold, from 5 percent up to 31 percent, were students were displaying unrealistically high levels of expectations that could not possibly be fulfilled, but would instead lead to a recipe for serious future disappointments.

A comprehensive study conducted in 2006 by the US National Research Consortium of Counselling Centres In Higher Education, found that in its study of over 15,000 college undergraduates with an average age of 22, 18 percent had seriously contemplated suicide and a shocking 8 percent had attempted it at some stage or other during their young lives.

With statistics like these, it is not hard to see that we as a society are failing our youth and ourselves. And that this modern world we are creating is clearly headed in the wrong direction. Unless there is a radical change in modern behaviours many young people will end up with serious emotional problems, mental illnesses and an increase in physical diseases they can cause.

Another study by a team at the University Of Toronto and published in the journal Cancer, showed the strong physical connection between emotional stress and physical disease. It suggested that children and adolescents who are physically abused have a 49 percent higher chance of developing cancer in adulthood.

And as adults, do we fare any better from the effects of stress ? Well many Western studies are now being conducted which certainly make you want to stop sharply, think deeply and re-assess your emotional life and health. When you suffer stressful emotions you don't just feel pain as you go through them, but the physical damage being caused runs deep and is storing up real and sometimes fatal illnesses for your future as well. From uncomfortable illnesses like skin problems, hair loss, tiredness and digestive disorders to the more life threatening conditions of heart diseases and cancers.

A study from a team at the Indiana University reported in the journal Cancer, reviewed data on 3.8 million people between 1973 and 2004. It found those who were married had a 65 percent chance of surviving cancer after 5 years, compared to a 45 percent chance of survival for those who were separated. The researchers commented that the stress of a break up and absence of a supportive partner most likely affected survival rates.

Researchers at the University of Chicago conducted a study of mice which were genetically predisposed to develop breast cancer. They found that socially isolated mice, living without the company of others, caused the speed and growth of their tumours to significantly increase. The scientists suggested that the same outcomes of the study would be produced in the human population.

A study by a team at the Karolinska Institute in Sweden found that being married or having a loving partner by middle age reduced your chance of developing dementia by nearly half. Whereas divorcees who did not remarry trebled their risk of dementia in later life. The study was based on 1,449 people.

Another study on 823 senior citizens in the US reported in the Archives Of General Psychiatry, found that those who were seen to be in the loneliest 10 percent category, were twice as likely to develop Alzheimer's.

Researchers found that those who reported the most negative aspects in their personal relationships, amongst a group of 9000 men and women in the UK, had a 34 percent increased risk of heart disease. As published in the Archives Of Internal Medicine.

A team from the University Of British Columbia reviewed 26 separate studies involving over 9000 patients and concluded that in cancer patients, death rates were 39 percent higher in those who were diagnosed with depression. As featured in the journal Cancer.

Researchers at the Ben-Gurion University found a clear link between breast cancer and outlook in their study, as published in the Journal BMC Cancer. They found that women who had two or more personal crisis or tragedies in their lives were nearly two thirds more likely to develop breast cancer than the average woman. And furthermore the group who were most optimistic were 25 percent less likely to develop it.

Chapter Sixty Eight - Positive Versus Negative Emotions.

Up until now we have mainly discussed negative emotions and their effects in the body and the mind. We have looked at the way fear, stress, anger, over excitement, loneliness, grief, sadness, frustration, nervousness, anxiety, shock, irritability, worry, sorrow, tension, depression, disappointment, despair and so on, can all impede and damage your organs and even drain your levels of energy, blood and hormones. Practically all of them will wreak havoc on your system in large quantities or can drain and weaken it in smaller ones over a period of time.

Your mind too can be heavily burdened by these emotions, many of them such as anger, anxiety and fear prevent you from seeing clearly. They often cloud the mind, stopping it from thinking straight and finding solutions to problems. This can cause you to become trapped in a vicious circle, where your mind can become filled with irrational thoughts and behaviour, causing you more problems and difficulties, rather than helping you to get out of whatever trouble you have found yourself in. Everyone has had the experience of saying or doing things out of character during angry hot headed arguments, which are often regretted afterwards when things have cooled and calmed down. Or when the mind is struck by a bout of nerves and all it seems to be able to deliver is a bunch of seemingly dumb and even incomprehensible statements. Quite often many of our emotions seem to be more of a hindrance rather than a help to us.

However, there are a few emotions which do the opposite, rather than tightening and constricting flow through the organs and body, they relax and calm it, rather than burning up or draining the life force from you they gently stimulate and circulate it. Rather than creating pressure, harassing or dumbing your mind, they open it. Feeding it with power and energy to provide clarity, positivity and good judgement.

These emotions are simply unconditional love and happiness. They cause no negative restrictions in the body but instead invigorate and enliven it. Under their influence, your Qi moves smoothly and freely. Your resources are less used and required, leaving you with an abundance of blood and its nutrients. And your Jing essence remains untapped, slowing your aging and keeping your reserves of life enhancing hormones in good supply. You will find too, that the more you are in these states, the more your mind remains calm, cool, focused and clear headed, no matter what it is presented with. Thus giving it the best possible opportunity it has to rationally think its way, not just out of a problem, but also how it can create any light and positivity and gain any benefit out of a bad situation. How it can find the silver lining in a dark cloud.

Even in Western science they are beginning to understand the benefits of positivity and happiness to not just increasing value in the emotional life of an individual but also in strengthening and enhancing their physical health too.

Researchers from the Carnegie Mellon University, interviewed 334 people for a study. They assessed the emotional attitudes of each participant, placing them into either a positive or negative category, they then infected the subjects directly with Rhinovirus to cause them colds. In the positive group, those who developed colds had significantly fewer signs and symptoms than those who had been placed in the negative group.

US researchers, who studied the health of 1,700 people over a ten year period, placed the participants on a five point scale, according to their levels of happiness, joy and contentment. Those who were filled with stress and hostility placed at the low end of the scale. It was noted, that for each rise of one in the happiness scale, there was a 22 percent lower risk of developing heart disease. As reported in the European Heart Journal.

According to the Netherlands Institute Of Mental Health, their study which followed 545 men between the ages of 64 to 84 for 15 years, showed that those who had a positive, optimistic outlook on life, were 50 percent less likely to die from heart disease.

A study at the Mayo Clinic in the US involving 1,100 patients over a thirty year period, revealed that people with a positive optimistic outlook lived on average 19 percent longer than those who were pessimistic.

Researchers from Yale University, found that participants in their study which measured positive perceptions of aging over a 23 year period, concluded that those with the most positive attitudes outlived those with negative ones by an extra 7.5 years.

Chapter Sixty Nine - So What Can We Do ?

We have now seen how our insides, from the neck down, can starve our brains of essential supplies of blood, oxygen, energy and hormones that they need to function healthily. Or how they can overwhelm the brain, sending heat, phlegm and pressure into it and overfilling it with toxins. In either case the brain will be unable to function with clarity and full intelligence and therefore unable to come to proper solutions and conclusions to emotional problems.

We have also seen how the brain can perceive events from the external world, causing it to suffer and cause a vicious chain of events throughout the body leading to both more physical ailments and further mental and emotional ones too.

In order to resolve and prevent problems coming from the mind and emotions, we need to confront this issue through two separate ways.

Firstly, we can follow all the other methods that we have learnt in this book to keep our physical organs and their vital substances in as peek condition as possible. By doing this, the mind will be running on premium levels of energy and nutrients, giving it the best possible chance to stay strong, think clearly and with ease in any difficult circumstance.

Secondly, we can learn how to retrain our minds, through methods such as meditation, positive affirmations and awareness. These will all have dramatic impacts on restructuring our emotional characteristics. Weakening or even dissolving the negative emotions and empowering the positive useful life enhancing ones. These methods make us true masters of our own minds, bodies, lives and destinies.

The following chapters will begin to give us the mental tools necessary to begin this journey to a better existence, helping to free us from the prison of past troubling memories and enabling us to avoid any future assault from the outside world.

Chapter Seventy   -   The Power Of The Mind.

For thousands and thousands of years in both Eastern and ancient medicines from around the rest of the world, the power of the mind has been seen as an incredibly potent and powerful force. It has the ability, through the medium of suggestion and belief to make the body strong and healthy or the body weak and sick.

In the East, methods of mastering, manipulating and controlling the conscious and subconscious minds have been written into their medicines since their formations. From mantras to meditations to Shen Gong. Mind work is truly one of the great pillars supporting the foundations of Eastern medicine.

One of the best ways to increase your physical and mental health is to simply train your mind into a state of positivity, where all your internal reactions, such as the building of cells, and all your external communications, such as interactions with people and in general, are performed at peak and productive levels. Ensuring that when you are giving your best in a situation, in most cases that is what will be returned to you.

You could imagine that if you have the opposite, a negative depressed mind, your body will slump and feel tired. Everything from your concentration to your digestion will become sluggish. And even the reproduction of your cells will be less efficient, causing weaker cells to be created, which in turn will cause you to slump even further and lay the grounds for possible future illnesses.

Or say you are in work when you are feeling down, you may be too tired to be productive and get a job completed. Or your colleagues may not want to interact with you as they themselves don't want their own mood to be pulled down with negativity. This in turn may create a vicious circle causing you further practical work problems or feelings of isolation and more emotional pain.

So in real terms, the mind can have a strong impact on the physical, emotional, spiritual, and energetic bodies and also on the creation of positive or negative actual life events and situations surrounding it.

The Placebo Effect.

In Western Medicine and science, this physical effect is portrayed very clearly through the effects of placebo and nocebo. They are like a big pink elephant sitting in the corner of the room, creating problems for drug makers and putting a massive dent in the foundations of Western Medicine. Which unfortunately, has denied and ignored the effects and power of the mind throughout most of its existence.

Placebo is used in clinical drug and surgery trials, where a fake dummy pill is tested against a real medication to see if it has a genuine ability to heal or treat an illness. If a drug outperforms a placebo then it can be marketed. The problem for Western Medicine and drug makers, is that when you give sick people fake pills, that do absolutely nothing in the body, it has been found to cure them of their ills in about 30 percent of cases.

To spell this out clearly, the mind having believed it ingested a real active medicinal cure, but in reality a useless fake pill, enacted everything necessary in the body to cure it of an infliction, all by itself. The mind through the power of its own beliefs healed the body.

Every clinical trial that has been performed has noted a substantial placebo effect. It has even been shown in studies that when people are given two pills instead of one, there is a stronger effect and when dummy pills have been printed with a well known drug name they work even more effectively.

In a study by the Garvan Institute Of Medical Research, athletes were given a dummy pill, but were told it was a stimulant, a human growth hormone, used to build muscle and enhance speed and agility. After monitoring these athletes, there was a 3.5 to 7.5 percent improvement noted in their performance.

A study by scientists at Turin University gave 11 patients with Parkinson's disease real injections to temporarily relieve symptoms of muscle stiffness and tremors. They later gave the same patients a placebo without any medication and noticed that six of the 11 patients had decreases in rigidity and tremors. These patients also clearly showed a reduction in nerve cell activity in a part of the brain which is affected and damaged by Parkinson's disease.

A Paper in the Journal Of The National Cancer Institute reported a study by Mount Sinai School Of Medicine of 200 women with breast cancer. It showed that patients who had been hypnotized needed less anaesthetic and felt less pain, tiredness and nausea after surgery. Another study by Beth Israel Deaconess Medical Centre in the US, showed similar results concerning surgical operations and hypnosis.

Hypnosis is not a placebo but does clearly demonstrate the power of the mind. An interesting recent case concerned an overweight woman from England who travelled to a clinic in Spain. She was then put into a hypnotic state, and talked step by step through the procedure for gastric bypass surgery, a severe solution to weight loss. Now she did not actually get physical surgery, but her brain was fooled into believing she had. As a result she lost four stone in weight, a similar equivalent to what she would have lost if she had actually undergone real surgery.

In 1999 a UK Biotech firm testing their new vaccine for food allergies were very impressed by the strong results they received in their clinical trials, suggesting a high success rate of 75 percent.

That is until the results of the corresponding placebo trial came in, this fake dummy pill too delivered a 75 percent success rate. The new drug was inevitably scrapped.

To further compound the strength of the minds beliefs is the nocebo effect. With the nocebo effect, people taking fake pills often develop side effects associated with similar real pills. Symptoms such as burning sensations, sleepiness, fatigue, stomach problems, skin rashes, vomiting, weakness, dizziness, diarrhoea and swelling are often reported. Even such effects as tinnitus, loss of libido and upper respiratory tract infections. Most disturbingly are cases of patients given the wrong diagnosis of terminal illnesses. One such incident of an American patient who was wrongly told he had only months to live, duly died in the allotted time frame. The autopsy showed he was misdiagnosed and had no explanation as to why he died. Other studies have shown that patients who believe they will not survive surgery are far more likely to die during it. Research showed that women who believed they were particularly prone to heart attacks are nearly four times as likely to die from them. Even more than 50 percent of cancer patients start to experience nausea from taking chemo drugs days before the drugs could cause that actual effect in the body.

Eastern doctors are not however the only ones to notice the power of placebo. In a recent nationwide survey in the US of 1,200 internists, reported in the journal BMJ, it was found that nearly two thirds of them believed in prescribing placebos to treat patients with real ailments, and nearly half of them every month will prescribe placebos during their work. These doctors prescribed sedatives, vitamins, pain relievers, antibiotics and ineffectively small doses of drugs knowing that these pills would only produce placebo effects. Studies and polls carried out in Denmark, Britain and Sweden have all provided similar results to this US one, that many Western doctors believe in the power of the mind, something that they have not learnt from their Western medical textbooks and training.

And even though, it has been established that the majority of Western doctors believe in the mind and placebo, it is often routinely dismissed by Western Medicine. Some Western doctors and academics don't like to feel that their medicine could be in any way inadequate and missing such a key foundation. So foolishly from pride, they continue to ignore it and keep the status quo. If accepted it would clearly have massive implications and ramifications across the whole face of Western Medicine, and many Eastern medicines and some alternative ones would suddenly be given a credibility that would challenge the old established authority self proclaimed by Western Medicine. On top of that there would be serious financial implications, if you teach people how to heal and help themselves through the power and abilities contained in their own minds, then there will be less use for medicines, costly surgical procedures and screenings.

The more the mind focuses on something, the more it creates and grows it. Think for example of a toothache or other pain. The more you think of it the worse it seems to throb or ache. Whereas when the mind is distracted, by something you do or by someone around you, then the more the pain seems to diminish. Often nearly completely fading and disappearing into the background.

Bear this in mind the next time you watch an advert, read a leaflet or see a poster for a drug or medical condition. Or even when you sit down to watch an exciting, entertaining hospital or doctor related drama on your television. Taking messages from these commercials and programs can interfere with your subconscious, possibly planting negative suggestions there to recreate the conditions it has been fed. When we are surrounded by images and news of sickness, then we end up expecting to get sick, and once we do that, our minds are surely playing a significant role in its creation.

So we have two choices, we can induce our own placebo effect, encouraging positive thoughts and beliefs of love, happiness and abundant health. We can choose to see the good and positive around us, and when it is not there to sow seeds to create it. When we master this, our subconscious will respond by keeping our systems and physical bodies running in top health and peak condition.

Or we can dwell in the negative, we can complain and whinge and see the worst in everything and everyone, to see only the dark side of life, but by doing this, it is most likely we will create our own nocebos and self fulfilling prophecy of the pain and suffering attached to them. Our subconscious mind directed and filled with such gloom will listen deeply to this message and respond by creating and producing weakness and inevitably illness throughout our systems.

Chapter Seventy One - The Physical Mind.

Physically the brain is the centre of a collection of billions of inter connected nerve cells that run the bodies electrical networks, controlling activities and movements throughout the system. These electrical pathways, just like the rest of the body can be affected by simple factors. Such as too much heat, cold, dryness, dampness, phlegm or toxins.

When things become too hot, the mind can become over active, hyper and wound up. Physically the heat can expand blood and tissues, leading to pain and pressure, or even if it becomes too intense, to internal breakages and cellular damage.

When things are too cold, the mind loses its power and energy, thoughts and processes slow down and may get stuck, leading to poor concentration, memory and thought processes, and to low moods.

If things become too dry, cells won't be fed and nourished, and movement and thoughts becomes slow and grinding.

If they are the opposite, too damp, the mind can become blocked and bloated, leading to cloudy thinking, poor judgement and even dull heavy headaches. If any of these factors are prolonged, it can lead to mental illnesses and poor judgment and functioning, producing diseases like senility in old age.

Obviously to keep our brains physically healthy, we need to keep everything in balance and also to do the same things as needed to keep our bodies healthy.

We need moderate amounts of exercise to keep good blood flow through the thousands of miles of blood vessels in our brains. And also to keep our hearts strong, so they can pump proper amounts of blood and oxygen into the mind.

We need enough sleep to give our brains a rest and prevent information overwhelming and overloading them. Also during the night hormones will be released to repair and boost brain cells and their functioning.

And we need deep, strong healthy breathing to supply a plentiful quantity of energy producing oxygen to our minds. Practicing abdominal and complete breathing will provide this.

The other major physical way we affect our brains and their thinking is through diet. Toxic foods such as sugars, fats and processed oils and foods can all lead to phlegm congesting the mind and blocking it up. This often leads to poor mental functioning and illness.

Heating foods such as spices, alcohol, coffee and too much red tea can burn up phlegm, congealing it and making it more rank and toxic. Heat by itself can burn away nutrients supplying brain cells and over time, these starving cells may weaken and die.

Whereas too much cold and damp producing foods, such as physically cold meals and drinks, too much vegetables and sweet fruits like bananas, can steal the brains energy and cause fluids to accumulate there, giving you dull thinking and poor focus and memory.

Overall, for brain health, just like you would do for your body, keep your diet balanced against whatever conditions you find yourself in.

Some particular useful foods to support, nourish and keep the brain generally healthy are …

Unprocessed plant and fish oils, these help to encourage smooth and easy movement through the brain.

Bitter green tea, fruit and juices which unclogs the brain, clearing it of excess fluid, phlegm, toxins and heat.

Rice which provides energy and power for cells.

And small amounts of stimulants such as alcohol and spices, which can enliven your mind and spirit if energy levels have dropped too low.

Foods that are involved in the production of cell restoring and rejuvenating hormones are very helpful too, such as nuts, seeds, cinnamon, salt and mushrooms.

Chapter Seventy Two - The Thinking Mind.

The mind can be split into two basic areas that produce thoughts. They are the conscious and the subconscious minds.

The conscious mind, is the part of you that is reading and processing this sentence right now. It thinks, computes, makes judgements and decisions. It is active when we are awake and tries to make sense of the world we live in. It is fed information externally from society and its surroundings and internally from your soul. It has incredible power through focus, concentration and repetition to establish programs to run in your subconscious.

Whereas the conscious mind is more like the central processing unit of a computer, the subconscious is more like the programs that run on it and the data and information contained in the memory. The subconscious contains all the patterns, habits and routines originally formed at birth to run your body. And formed after that through your life experiences and programming from society. These programs help you run your body and your life on auto pilot, so your conscious mind is freed up to interact with new developments.

This is just like learning to drive a car, when you start to learn how to drive, your mind is very aware and notices every little action. However after a while, your subconscious having created patterns from repeated actions, takes over and you seem to be able to drive with ease. Your conscious mind is freed up and you can hold a conversation, listen to the radio, think of what you have to do later, and of course drive safely all at the same time.

Most of our reactions to life, come from our subconscious. Even when we meet new people or do new things, references from past experiences come constantly from the subconscious into the conscious mind, prompting us to behave in certain ways in these new situations. The problem is a lot of these prompts may not be beneficial or desirable. We may have lots of unwelcome habits now hardwired into our subconscious from negative past experiences we have endured. These may now continually prompt us to behave in sad, angry, shy, anxious, critical or fearful ways and so on. We may even make judgements about people and situations not on the real current events and facts we are presented with, but on pre-judgements formed by past memories in our subconscious. This is obviously not sensible or productive in leading us towards healthy and happy lives. And often instead traps us into behaviour which prolongs misery and suffering.

The other common action the subconscious takes, is to feed the conscious mind with whatever predominant emotions it has learnt to have most of. This means that if it has mainly been fed sadness and negativity, then even when it experiences something joyous, it quite often and quickly returns to what it knows most of, in this case negativity.

The good news is that if we consistently practice optimism, positivity and healthy mental outlooks, then that is what our subconscious will eventually push forth. When it reaches this state then even if we are currently going through a bad experience, if our subconscious has been formed with positive thoughts it will be pushing that into our minds, buoying and strengthening them up and helping us to calmly and more easily think our way through whatever it is we are facing.

We will talk more about the many positive things we can do to influence and retrain our subconscious minds shortly.

However I must emphasize that with any of these methods or ones for other health improvements described earlier in the book, that they must initially be constantly reinforced and practiced. New programs and habits must be reiterated over and over again in the subconscious, until they rewrite whatever negative pattern of behaviour you are trying to change. After that they should be constantly topped up through methods such as meditation, positive affirmations and right thinking.

Become The Observer.

With the mind you must become its observer. You must watch and take note of thoughts and emotions as they come up into the brain. Objectively start to judge them and their reactions throughout you and your body. And see if they are useful to you or not. Are they genuine or just repetitive behaviour from what your subconscious has been conditioned to believe.

Examine all the emotions as they appear, think about them logically and rationally. For example, if we think about anger, do you really want to be controlled by it or have to deal with the pain it brings you. In nearly all cases it won't lead to the best outcome in an argument, instead it quite often leads you to say and do things you would not if you had stayed cool and clearheaded. Later you will most likely start to regret, wishing you could take back what you had said. Or how about its effect on the other person, getting them all riled up and aggressive as well. Now two minds are acting irrationally and all common sense and reasoning disappears. Instead if you stay calm and focused you will find your mind can logical think its way out of a problem and come up with the best solution for all involved.

However, anger is not alone, most emotions, be they sadness, guilt, fear, jealousy, bitterness, disappointment or the like, only produce negative consequences and detrimental effects, for both you and those who are around you. Examine them all, and one by one let all the negative ones go from your life. Leaving you to embrace the only ones that actually help your body in a positive way, the emotions of happiness and love, they are the only ones you truly want or need.

Memories quite often have emotions attached to them. For example you will have many of them lodged in your brain that make you angry when you think of them. You could pay a psychiatrist a fortune to sit with you and talk you through resolving each one of them. It would also be a very painful and disturbing experience as each old memory is rehashed and felt again. But if you change the big picture. If in this case you resolve and change your beliefs regarding anger and its validity, then you will find all past memories tainted by anger begin to diminish, leaving only the lesson to be learned and the wisdom garnished from that memory left behind.

Be Careful What You Feed Your Mind.

When you sit down to watch television tonight or even start to read a novel, be careful what you have chosen to take in. Our modern society constantly pushes drama and excitement towards us. There are very few family orientated, heart warming and positive programs anymore. Instead we have ones filled with violence, sadness, cheapened and exploitive sex, wealth and greed, corruption, gossip, betrayal and many other negative aspects and emotions. Unfortunately when we are watching these, particularly if we start to get emotionally involved, our subconscious starts to absorb this presentation as if we are part of it. If we constantly watch or read about sadness our minds will become more depressed, if we watch violence we will feel more violent, if we watch programs about gossip, we will be encouraged to talk negatively about others and so forth.

So when your are watching TV, reading or even hanging out with friends, be careful what is being fed into your subconscious as this is what will be projected into your life. Just as you watch your diet and avoid eating too much junk food, be just as careful in preventing junk from being fed to your mind and soul. Instead choose more uplifting and positive TV and books to read. If you are around negative people, those who gossip, whinge and constantly complain, then push the conversation to more positive topics. You too should avoid complaining and gossiping as well as this is only encouraging and feeding a negative state in your own mind and leading you further away from your goal of happiness.

Dealing With Negativity And Painful Past Experiences.

Unfortunately in life, bad things can happen to both good and bad people. Those who do wrong and create pain for others, have no one to blame but themselves when inevitably the consequences of their own actions come back to their doorstep. But for those who practice good and do no harm, life can sometimes seem very unjust and unfair. We can regularly meet selfish, inconsiderate, thoughtless and corrupt people. Sometimes in our families, relationships, co-workers, strangers and even sometimes friends who can abuse our trust and let us down and turn out to be anything but friendly.

When something bad happens to us, especially in childhood when our minds have less wisdom and experience, our subconscious often reacts to pain by trying to build a wall around our emotional hearts and souls to protect them. We end up pushing this part of us deeper and deeper inside, disconnecting it from the cruel behaviours of some other humans. The problem is, when we close our souls off, we are also closing off the ability to feel and surround ourselves in the only real and meaningful love and happiness that there is to be found in our lives. If we have not access to our souls then we can never truly feel or know what real love is.

The outside world is quite good at feeding us with pleasure. However these temporary highs and fixes often only numb our pain and distract our minds from our real issues. Leaving us back in the same spot and facing the same problems we originally had when the pleasure has passed. On the other hand, if we can manage to take down the walls around our hearts and souls, then as we feed them with positivity and real wisdom, they will grow and we will find that a genuine love comes forth from them, that keeps us protected and on a continuous high.

Unless you are well versed in the wisdom of enlightenment or have been lucky enough to have developed real depth and wisdom through your own experiences, this type of love is very difficult to describe and understand. The love that comes from the soul is a true and genuine sense of happiness and belonging. It is more of a feeling than a thought. It is warm, comforting, secure, peaceful and yet at the same time alive and invigorating. It is very unlike pleasure, which is a purely mental experience, giving you a boost and then dropping you, often leaving you disappointed and in a state of craving for a new experience to replace it. That is not real happiness. Not even close.

The love emitted from the soul is entirely independent of all external forces outside the human being, it does not require wealth, power, vanity or any of the other trappings of the ego to produce it. This type of love is the exact thing that all human beings need to complete and fulfil their existence. Unfortunately, most people who get caught up in the consumerism and competition of our modern capitalistic world, are searching for this happiness but are looking entirely in the wrong places where it cannot be found. Instead of outside, we need to turn our focus back inside and release our souls.

This love inside is free and abundant. It takes nothing from you to create it but in turn relaxes and empowers you. Your physical health and mental well being will thrive on it. It makes you smile, gives you bliss, makes you feel great, with it you often find you are happy for no reason at all. It has no limits. The closer you get to real love in the soul, the closer you get to long fulfilling happiness, to creating your own personal heaven on earth.

But to do this, it takes you to free your soul, to allow it to come back out into this sometimes harsh world. This time however, to protect your sensitive soul, unlike when you were a child and everything you experienced got dumped into your subconscious, this time using proper mental techniques and awareness, you will be in control and choose not only what is now allowed into your mind, but you will also reprogram what is already there. Clearing away any negative emotions and past traumatic experiences which are still repeating on your conscious mind and interfering with your present day happiness.

To remove the power attached to these past negative memories we must diminish any emotion attached to them. By altering our beliefs and views regarding emotions at the higher level, this will automatically start to reduce undesirable emotions from our memories.

But in this process, we should definitely garnish any wisdom or lesson to be learnt from a past experience, as this will help us to make better choices in our present. From bad events we should learn and become wise, otherwise we are bound to make similar mistakes again and trap ourselves in a cycle of suffering.

We also need to forgive others in order to release ourselves from the past. This does not mean that we excuse their behaviour, it just means we lose the hate and the anger. For those emotions are imprisoning us and preventing us from moving on.

If you are someone who has harmed others in the past and you are filled with guilt and shame, then you too need to let these go. It is a good thing that you feel bad for what you have done. It shows that you are sorry and have begun to take responsibility for your actions. So once you have learnt and grown from any past mistake, once you are now committed to positive change and will do your best to avoid repeating any problems you may have caused, then you have now become a different person, a new you. Your mind and soul are no longer forming the same person who harmed others. Your soul has matured and developed. So it is time to forgive yourself, move on and create a wiser happier future for yourself and all others who become a part of it.

Chapter Seventy Three   -   More Positive Stuff To Do.

Smile - Smile meaningfully as much as possible. And even when you don't want to smile, smile anyway. A smile ignites electrical pathways in the brain which cause a calming and uplifting effect throughout the body. Every time you smile you are benefiting your physical body and health. In the same way, hold your posture upright and open. This too, sends signals to the subconscious that all is well and good. In this state of mind, the subconscious will carry out tasks around the body in peak performance, rather than being sluggish and disruptive.

Breathe - By having an open posture it will also enable you to breathe properly. Remember to breathe slowly and deeply, this will energize both body and mind, powering up your spirit and strengthening your positive emotions. Without breath, oxygen in the brain is reduced and it will most likely falter and panic, increasing your worries and problems.

One of the first things to be affected when you get stressed is your breathing, as your body tenses, the muscles around your ribcage seize and prevent you from inhaling properly. So consciously be aware of this and practice daily breathing techniques to re-enforce good breathing behaviour. This is important for everyone to do, but is especially important for anyone who works behind a desk or at a computer.

Negative Chat - Cut out the pessimism, gossip and defeatist self talk. All these are sending very negative messages to your subconscious and will corrupt it, causing it to create poor health and even more problems in your life. Statements like, "I can't" and "it's too difficult" re-enforce weak patterns of thinking and will lead you away from your goals.

Always practice optimism and keep your mind positive. Look on the bright side of life. Look for the opportunities, not the problems.

Your subconscious mind grows and creates more of anything it dwells on. It does not make logical decisions but merely follows suggestions from the conscious mind. If you say think of a red balloon, you will see an image of a red balloon pulled from your subconscious memory banks in to your mind. However if you say the opposite, don't think of a red balloon, you will still get the same result. So always concentrate on what you do want rather than on what you want to avoid or else the subconscious will just start to produce the very things you are trying to escape from.

If you consciously dwell on negativity, your subconscious will look for events within and outside of you to create more of the same. So always look for, embrace and re-enforce positivity, in your words, in your thoughts and in your actions. Otherwise your negativity will just create a self fulfilling prophecy and bring you more of its kind.

This is one of the reasons why everyone should practice being good, because when you are concentrating on being mean or bad, in actuality you are focusing that state into your subconscious mind and it will inevitably do its best to create the same state for you that you have been creating for others. Only good sincere thoughts can manifest and bring to you the real happiness you truly long for.

By practising and being loving, peaceful and positive this will eventually become the natural state inside your mind. However, be positive but be wise. Do not tolerate bad situations or people. Don't get dramatic or angry, just smarten up and move on. Take your business and kindness elsewhere, where it and you can be respected and appreciated.

Visualize Happiness - Don't just look for the positive side to an event but actively create and imagine a joyous outcome in your mind. This will get your subconscious to work in the background to find ways to accomplish this goal. It may subtlety make you behave in a different manner or push you to make a different intuitive choice to accomplish this outcome. It is much more logical to have it visualizing happiness and creativity, and working with your consciousness, rather than having it caught up in some form of negative learned past behaviour, which could only lead to problems for you.

Lose The Fight, The Resistance, The Anger - This pattern accomplishes nothing and only causes destruction. If there is a negative outcome it often makes it harder to swallow and more damaging to the body and the mind. Better to keep tranquil, which will allow your mind to act in the clearest and most logical manner, in order to attain the achievement you want.

In the East there are many old sayings about this. They say it is better to be like a soft blade of grass than a hard tree in a storm. The blade of grass bends back and forth under the force of the gale and survives, whereas the solid tree stands firm but then often finds its branches or trunk broken by this behaviour.

So better to stop fighting every little thing in life that does not go your way. Be sure to stay true to your inner self and keep your goals and beliefs, but do change paths and move around the obstacles that life throws in front of you, rather than trying to fight them all. You will accomplish much more in the long run, save yourself lots of energy and avoid much frustration and heartache by following this approach.

Live In The Present - Create a positive mentality, then live in the now. Enjoy the moment, the happiness and love you are creating right now. When you do things for others, forget thoughts of any future reward or compensation for what you are giving them. Lose the expectations and instead live in the love and happiness you are generating right now. That is your reward, you are already there, your happiness is already complete, enjoy it.

Free Yourself And Embrace Happiness In Any Form - Stop conforming to what society tells you is hip, trendy and cool. Make up your own mind up and stop listening to others. The object of life is to become happy, not to listen to the mindless who are just following the crowd. Clearly as rates of anxiety and depression are dramatically increasing, it is very unwise to simply follow the crowd anymore, unless you too want to end up becoming sick and unhappy.

I wasted considerable amounts of my younger life trying to live up to the expectations of others and there often ill formed and poorly thought out ideologies. So break free, start enjoying what you want, not what is merely fashionable and correct in society. The next time you buy something, buy it because you like it, because its colour, its texture, its shape makes you interested in it and makes you smile, not because someone has told you this will keep your standing in society as one of the trendy people.

The next time you make friends with someone, do it because you like them, not because they are the coolest people to hang with and will make you look good in front of your peers. Be friends with them because they are nice, they are good people and forget what ranking society has given them. So many good relationships and opportunities for happiness have been destroyed because one person did not think it was cool to hang around another. As young kids we did not care what our friends looked like or the way they acted. We only cared about having fun with them. It was only after being bullied by society that we changed our minds. So break free and get that genuineness back into your relationships. And you will find plenty of real love and happiness comes along with it too.

Remember, health and happiness are your goals. It is not necessary to become wealthy and successful, but only to become healthy and happy. It is not necessary to become famous and popular, but only to become healthy and happy. Always keep this thought active and conscious in your mind. Follow it and you will be truly rewarded.

Do The Groundwork - You get back what you give. So if you want real, honest, good rewarding relationships. Then expect to put in some real effort to build up trust and strong foundations in them. If you do encourage and create genuine friendships and relationships, you will be rewarded with so much more than money can buy you. And if you stumble upon genuinely good and enlightened people, people who are wised up and understand about love, life and goodness, then treat them well and hold onto them. For they are worth more than their weight in gold and will give you back far more than you could possibly have imagined.

Spend less of your time watching TV and on the internet and more of your time building honest, good, loving, real relationships that will carry you with a smile on your face and love in your heart into a beautiful and peaceful old age. You will have spent your entire life being happy and loving. And if there is an afterlife, such a beautiful soul you have created will truly be embraced.

Do Good, Spread Love - By practising good and promoting love, peace, happiness, honesty, wisdom, meaning and joy, we start a chain reaction of positive actions around us that will feed into society. The more we promote this, the more good will return to us and enhance our own lives. But if we promote criticism, gossip, judgement, bitterness, sourness, selfishness, then the odds are that is what will be returned to us.

You cannot go wrong by dwelling on love, peace and happiness. Focus on them to bring more of the same into your life.

"Thousands of candles can be lit from a single candle, and the life of the candle will not be shortened, happiness never diminishes by being shared" - Buddha.

Chapter Seventy Four - Mastering The Mind.

Meditation is a method used to cultivate energy, to gain control of and master the subconscious mind, and then to harness this energy and clear thinking to eventually lead the mind towards enlightenment.

The first step is to gather energy and master the subconscious. The subconscious is like a storehouse of past experiences, memories and their attached emotions. Using data it has acquired through life and its original programming past on from your parents and ancestors, it is in charge of running and maintaining all background functioning. Most of your daily experiences are not performed by your conscious mind but are run by your subconscious, leaving you in a state of running on auto pilot.

From the physical like your breathing, to automatic emotional responses pulled from past learned behaviour, to facial expressions and other habits and characteristics you have formed, to speaking in a foreign language or performing any other skill you have learnt. It is basically responsible for everything your conscious mind isn't directly participating in. And even the decisions you make consciously, are often strongly prompted from pre-formed judgements in the subconscious as opposed to open, fresh, re-examination of the current situation you are dealing with.

If you do not take full charge of your mind and instead let your subconscious take over and run the show, then many problems can start to surface. We have already seen how if our subconscious is in a negative state and running in a poor or dismal way, it clearly sends out orders that will produce lower quality functioning and regeneration in the physical body. If our subconscious is filled with bad experiences and stress, as it becomes more paralysed by detrimental emotions, it will also tighten and seize up movement and activity in the body causing the emergence of further physical ills.

Another set of problems can occur from our subconscious when it is overwhelmed by thoughts. The Chinese often then refer to it disrespectfully as the chattering monkey. It has become filled with too many worries, cares, emotions and problems. It simply becomes less productive and instead starts to flush gibberish and an abundance of thoughts into our consciousness. Which then, apart from the anxiety, cannot find the peace and clarity it needs to make the right decisions and steer its way out of life's problems.

Yet another malicious battle occurs between the ego, created by the subconscious and our true being, our souls. The ego is formed entirely in the subconscious mind. And is a projection of our self importance based upon observations and past experiences. The ego is always hungry and its desires can never be quenched, if one is fulfilled it is simply replaced by another, it always demands more and more, and to be better than others. It has no soul or values, it is artificial and purely influenced by external events in society. It is not useful to its owner, who it often leads in the wrong direction, dragging them into negativity, and stealing energy and attention from the real objectives in life. It can only create pleasure but not happiness. And detracts power and limelight away from the persons inner self, their soul.

Nor is it any use to the outside world. The ego spreads criticism, greed, gluttony, competition and other negative qualities. It favours no-one but itself. When it is winning the battle against the soul, the person will not have the opportunity to experience real happiness and love. But will be left on a pleasure seeking rollercoaster of emotional ups and downs. As time goes by, and the enemies of the ego, such as age and loss of power start to win, there inevitably comes the time when the downs greatly start to smother the ups, leading you into a life of bitter misery.

If you are to ever truly find happiness and the superior health and well being that thrives in that state, then at some stage you must deal with the ego in your subconscious, and quite simply diminish its power and destroy it.

Meditation, when practised correctly, can be a very successful method to master and control the subconscious mind and to quell the ego within it.

Types Of Meditation.

There are many methods and styles of meditation. When you study them, you begin to see clear patterns of their common threads. If you want you can sit cross legged in the Lotus position. Or you can adopt a pose from Yoga. Yoga is not just a set of stretching exercises as believed to be by many in the West, but is actually a spiritual practice. Yoga means union, and in this case to unify with God and the Universe. In the West, it is mostly practiced as a set of exercises with a little meditation thrown in. In the East, the opposite is true and with the exercises, just as in Qi Gong, there is a strong emphasis placed on gathering and manipulating energy through them.

My personal favourite form of meditation is through Qi Gong exercises. But if you are versed in Yoga or some other method then you can try incorporating some of the techniques shortly described into your own style of meditation.

If you are a strong follower of a particular religious faith, then do not think that by practising meditation you have aligned yourself with any other type of religion. Historically, in the Christian and other Western religions, meditation has always had a strong place. Nuns and monks have always followed a similar practice through everything from vows of silence and isolation, to prayer and meditation. They do this to find quiet and peace in their minds, to allow deeper clarity and connection with their souls and God. In the East, nearly every religion, be they Buddhist, Taoist, Hindu or so forth, uses meditation also for this exact same purpose. So do not have any fear that you are betraying your religion by following any of the meditative techniques in this book. They are just simply good techniques to allow you to have more control of your own mind. From this book you can take whatever techniques you find beneficial and apply them to your own religious beliefs.

If you are an atheist or have some other form of belief, meditation will also only benefit you, by increasing the energy and power in your brain, allowing it to function more calmly and clearly, and therefore helping you to make better and more productive decisions in your life, and thus allowing it to be more successful and fulfilling.

Chapter Seventy Five - Qi Gong.

In the simplest form, Qi means energy and Gong means work. Qi Gong is the art of cultivating energy. Its aim is to increase the amount of energy in the body, mind and spirit. This energy powers up all living parts, enhancing their functioning. This increased energy will further help to process food and air more effectively to help create more blood and nutrients to nourish and protect our physical bodies and calm and stimulate our minds. It will help to preserve cells, slow down ageing and increase general health and well being.

Qi Gong is thousands of years old and forms part of the roots and foundations of Chinese Medicine. One version of exercises is said to have been brought by Bodhidharma to the Shaolin Monastery in China to strengthen the monks there. Who by sitting still for long hours in meditation in the cold weather, had developed health problems from poor circulation. The standing and moving postures of Qi Gong alleviated any problems that may have come from seated meditations. It gave them superior energy and allowed them to live longer and have more time to generate spiritual wisdom and energies.

Qi Gong is historically used for three main areas, they are healing, martial arts and spiritual progression. In medicine it is used to build, heal and manipulate internal energies which control the physical body and mental and emotional welfare. In martial arts it is used to create power, speed, skill, agility, alertness and strength for combat. It also provides lots of power for superior ability to recuperate from any injuries. In spirituality it is used to gain control of the mind and then to flood it and the soul with energy to attain wisdom and enlightenment.

In China, it is estimated that up to 160 million Chinese people practise Qi Gong exercises every day. They are usually seen in parks first thing in the morning, before going off to work. There are many thousands of Qi Gong routines, such as Zhan Zhuang, a group of still postures used to gather energy and also for Shen Gong. Shen Gong is spirit and mind work practised during Qi gong. It is used in areas such as retraining the subconscious mind into more positive and life affirming beliefs. There are also moving postures such as the Ba Duan Jin, which help to stimulate and circulate energy through specific organs and pathways in the body.

By boosting and increasing energy, every single part of the body and mind are enhanced. With more energy, it is easier to think clearly and creatively. Mental capabilities such as concentration, memory, sharpness, thought processing and alertness are all improved. With a calmer, clearer and more stable mind, wisdom and awareness start to flourish. The ego is naturally reduced and the soul begins to take its true position as commander of the human vessel.

Its physical effects are numerous. With extra power in the organs, many weaknesses are brought back to strong activity, thus creating the power to heal any existing illnesses and problems. As cells are kept healthy and filled with energy, their natural deterioration slows down, diminishing the need for hormones to be used in boosting them up and therefore preserving Jing essence and slowing down aging. With stronger organs and more steady blood, nutrients, energy and oxygen reaching the mind, the mood too is stabilized and lifted. Giving a less stressful, calmer and happier life. In general, Qi Gong simply makes life easier and a whole lot more enjoyable and worth living.

How It Works.

Qi Gong charges and generates energy in our bodies through many different ways.

For starters there is the breathing technique used while practising. It is of course complete breathing, using both the lungs and abdomen to inhale, hold and push oxygen through our systems. Oxygen is energy and as it floods through our bodies and minds, it invigorates every living cell. It additionally allows our bodies to pull extra electrons through the air into them which further encourages and builds a healthy charge in our systems.

By deep breathing we are also cleansing toxins and carbon from our blood stream, this allows more energy to gather, as less power is required to push nutrients through and carry out functioning in an unpolluted less burdened system.

With the right posture, both energy and nutrients can also move and perform more effectively, thus again saving them from being needlessly used up and squandered. With Qi Gong postures, we are talking about opening up the circulatory system, the lymph system, the nervous system and also the energetic system, throughout the body and particularly along and around the spine.

Next up, we generate energy through a slight amount of tension as we hold our Qi Gong stance. This is the right amount of resistance to stimulate, strengthen and move our energy, but is not enough to start using it up and weakening it.

When we do normal exercises we start to feel hot as we increase our energy levels to perform whatever workout or activity we are attempting. Unfortunately, by the time the exercise is finished we have pushed ourselves too far and have used up all the energy that was created. This usually ends up leaving us feeling tired and depleted.

However, every time we have a Qi Gong session, we generate a smaller amount of energy, but in this case we keep it. And it slowly over repeated practice starts to accumulate in our bodies. After a time, we have built up enough energy to easily perform all our daily requirements and then also to have a back up reserve of energy, which can be used anytime we are threatened by external events, such as accidents, attacks by virus and bacteria, stressful situations, or even a particularly hard days work and so forth.

In yet another way, Qi Gong generates extra energy through controlling the mind and the emotions more efficiently. When our minds are quiet, relaxed and at peace, then the chattering monkey of your subconscious consumes far less energy. Freeing it up and letting the power flow out of the mind and into the body, where it can prop up your organs, allowing them to function more effectively and smoothly.

The more anxious and wound up your mind is, then the more uncontrolled thoughts flow back and forth from the subconscious and more energy will be wasted and burnt up. Particularly damaging are negative emotions which can easily eat up your power and drain you of life. Think of how tired and weak you feel after a shock or after an argument.

By using Qi Gong to quiet the mind and strengthen its ability to control emotions, you will find you have plenty of energy left for it to run better and also to increase health and strength in the rest of the body.

Finally, by removing those negative emotions and using meditations to replace them with positive ones, this will also give you a big energy boost. Think of how brimming with life and energy you are, when you feel happy and things are going well for you. Through Qi Gong you can manipulate the mind to induce this state at all times.

Chapter Seventy Six   -   The Energy Body.

Along with our physical body, our mental body composed of the conscious and subconscious minds, and our spirit body, we also have our energetic body. It is made from a series of energy pathways which flow throughout every part of our system, from our organs to our minds, feeding everywhere with power and life.

In the centre core of the body there is a beam of energy, referred to as the Taiji Pole, which runs from the top of our heads to beneath our groin. There are several pools of energy along this line, but in particular there are three very important ones, which act like reservoirs and storehouses to power the organs surrounding them. The Chinese refer to them as dantians, or in English, heavenly places.

Heavenly Places.

The lower dantian, is in the central line of the body, at the level just below the belly button. It is the largest pool of energy in most people and is of primary importance for maintaining and prolonging life. It can act like a spare set of batteries to power us up if we overextend ourselves. It provides back up power to two very important sets of organs in its immediate vicinity. The digestion which breaks down and absorbs our food to produce nutrients and more energy. And the kidneys and hormonal glands which maintain proper production and release of our Jing and hormones. Both these organs in health can give us strength and prolong our lives, or in disease and weakness can shorten them.

The middle dantian, located in the centre of our chest, is powering up our hearts, lungs and livers. These organs, as we have learnt, have strong implications for our emotional health and well being. If the power in these organs becomes weak or blocked then our minds and emotions become unstable and low. So this energy centre is strongly connected with maintaining and providing emotional and mental support in health, or instability in illness.

The upper dantian, is located inside the brain in the area behind the centre of the eyebrows. It obviously has a great impact on our mental intelligence and faculties, but is also related to our psychic and spiritual awareness.

Feeling Energy.

When performing Qi Gong it is very common to feel Qi. Especially if you have been practising for a while and have developed the ability to easily gather energy.

Qi often feels like a tingling warm sensation as it passes through and builds up in certain parts of your system.

There is a very simple exercise you can do to feel energy. It works very quickly for most people who try it.

To do the exercise, stand up straight in a warm, well ventilated room, and start to take long, slow, deep breaths. Then after a couple of minutes, bring your hands close together, and start to bring them very slowly in and out, without letting them touch each other. Continue to take long breaths, separating the hands as you breathe in and bringing them towards each other as you breathe out.

After a few minutes of this, most people will start to feel an invisible pressure beginning to build up between their hands. It sometimes feels like the way two magnets with the same magnetic poles being brought together invisibly force each other apart. Inside their hands, there may be feelings of tingling, pulsing, warmth or heat. The air between the hands may feel heavier and denser.

Now take one hand and hold it an inch or two above the other, then continue to breathe deeply and very slowly move your hand up and over your exposed arm. Again most people will feel sensations without it touching the bare skin on their arm. This is the Qi that they are feeling.

Chapter Seventy Seven - How To Do Qi Gong.

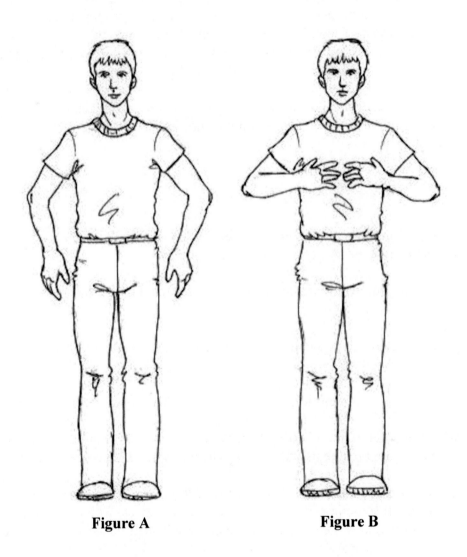

Figure A   **Figure B**

The Stance.

There are many different standing stances in Qi Gong. In this book we will concentrate on just two of them. For most people, they will get a very effective workout from just these two positions. The first is called Wuji (as shown in Figure A), and is probably the most well known Qi Gong posture.

It kind of resembles the pose a wild west gunslinger from an old cowboy movie would have made.

To form the stance …

1) Place your feet, with your toes pointed forwards, at roughly shoulder width apart.

2) Imagine there is a cord attached to the top of your head and it is pulling you upwards. Forcing you to stand as erect and as straight as possible.

The idea behind this is to open all the muscles along either side of the spine allowing circulation to move much more freely. It also relieves the pressure on the organs, created from poor posture and slouching positions. It opens the lungs and abdomen allowing you to breathe more easily and deeply. And it also aligns the energy pools through the centre line of the body.

3) To further facilitate a straight body and spine. Bend your knees slightly, an inch or two will suffice. And then pull your bottom a little bit forward. This straightens the lower part of your spine.

4) You will notice too that the back of your head juts out and breaks the straight alignment, so tilt your chin down about an inch, to reduce this bump.

5) Next open your chest and shoulders outwards towards your sides, but don't hunch them up. Keep the muscles relaxed but stretch out the skeletal structure.

6) Now imagine a baseball or an egg under each armpit, so they too are slightly opened.

7) Next hold your hands out about eight to twelve inches from your hips.

8) Imagine there is a marble between each finger, so they are held open as well. Neither allow them to touch each other nor stretch them too wide, just have them open in a middle position.

And that is it, your stance is complete.

This is the most basic standing pose and probably the best one all round. When you are in it, try to stay as still as you can, keep the pose open and wide but relax the muscles. Just like clothes lie on a hanger, allow your muscles to lie on your opened skeletal structure. Always try to perform abdominal and complete breathing while in this pose. Your body is open and correctly aligned, so it should be easy to perform from here.

The second stance is the same as the first one, except you hold your arms up at the level of your shoulders, (as shown in Figure B). You can imagine you are wrapping your arms around a giant beach ball. Sometimes it is referred to as hugging a tree, as you could visualize wrapping your arms around the trunk of a big old tree.

Make sure your elbows are slightly bent in this position. And align your fingertips up with each other. Create a circular space between your chest and arms, but don't allow your fingers to touch, instead keep them about eight to twelve inches apart.

Qi Gong is normally performed standing but if you are too weak or recovering from illness you can sit or even lie down and try to hold a similar posture from that position.

Preparation For Your Routine.

Try to find a quiet area where you won't be disturbed to do your practice. Outside in fresh clean air, with a plentiful supply of negatively charged ions is ideal, but it is ok to practice indoors too. However if you do, then open a window and let some air circulate in and around you. If the air is cold, be sure to wrap up well and keep yourself warm. Loosen your belt and try to wear loose unrestrictive clothing if you can.

As you will usually be standing in each Qi Gong pose for a set period of time, it is best to get yourself a watch or an alarm with some sort of count down timer on it. This is much better than having to keep distracting yourself by having to repeatedly check a clock to see when to switch poses and finish up the routine.

When you initially start Qi Gong, you might find it difficult to keep quiet or even be disturbed by the quiet itself. If this is the case you can have music playing softly in the background. But choose music that has no chorus or anything to sing along too, so the mind can't join in with it. Gentle classical music is often ideal as it distracts and leads the mind rather than allowing it to co-create the music.

The best and easiest time to practice Qi Gong is usually first thing in the morning. If you put it off until later in the day, you may often find you don't manage to get around to it, and the whole day slips by without your Qi Gong session. As Qi Gong gradually and slowly accumulates the energy in your body, it is essential to do it nearly every day to achieve positive productive effects. So getting your practice over and done with first thing in the morning is for most people the best way to keep to a steady routine and achieve this.

Chapter Seventy Eight - A Qi Gong Practice Routine.

There follows a simple easy to do yet very effective Qi Gong and meditation routine. It incorporates all major energetic, mental and spiritual work necessary for good health and happiness.

To start with assume the first posture that we learnt in the previous chapter. You can remain in this posture for the entire routine, or after a few minutes move into the second posture and stay in it until you have finished, or even you can swap back and forth between the two every few minutes. It is entirely up to you.

From there follow the next series of steps. You can use them as your guide, you don't have to be very strict and if you feel that a change would benefit you, then feel free to personalize it into your own version of the routine.

Step 1) Relax.

Breathe in, hold, then exhale and relax your mind and every other part of your body. Let all stress, worries and cares fade away and be released from your body, mind and soul. Starting at the top of your head, take in a deep breath and then relax each body part in turn.

Relax your facial muscles, your neck, shoulders, chest, back, abdomen, internal organs, arms, hands, buttocks, hips, thighs, calves and feet.

Sometimes people find it difficult to initially relax a muscle area. So you can start by doing the opposite to show you how. That is, gently tense the area, hold it, then loosen it and feel it soften and relax.

2) Complete Breathing.

Now start to take in deep abdominal and complete breaths, feeling the energy being pulled deep down into your lower belly. Do this for at least eight slow breaths.

At this point I need to start explaining a little bit about implanting suggestions into and leading the subconscious mind, before we continue with the routine.

To alter programs, behaviour and memories in our subconscious, we need to quieten and subdue it. The more we can turn it off, the more we can get it to listen to our suggestion. So just like in a hypnotic trance, try to go into a deep state of quiet and calmness. And turn off the chattering monkey. You will find that your conscious mind has a much stronger ability to implant suggestions into your subconscious in this state.

Through focusing we also strengthen our conscious mind, we empower it and give it control. Again enabling it to more successfully rewrite the subconscious mind. Anytime we focus on just one thing, such as breathing, a candle or a spot on the wall, then we are pushing energy into our conscious mind making it more powerful.

Next up we can use imagery, visualizations and word associations.

As we are living our lives, our subconscious is recording and interpreting everything in the fore and backgrounds. It starts to associate positivity with light, warmth, white, gold, sunshine, angels, heroes, success, health and happiness and so on. Negativity with darkness, cold, boredom, pain, sadness, demons and villains etc. So in our subconscious minds we have developed a history of good life affirming words and images. Things that will light up the subconscious, making it run well, producing health and joy in the body. And also negative soul destroying words and images, causing the subconscious to slow, falter and produce ill health. When we are practising Qi Gong, we should only encourage and utilize these positive images and word associations to emphasize our desired results to the subconscious. Quite often a striking image of health and power can have a greater more pronounced effect on the subconscious than just telling it to get healthy.

When you are meditating on words and images, make sure you attach positive happy emotions and feelings to them. If you were to send a message like, "I will have a successful interview tomorrow", while your feeling nervous and fearful, the subconscious will get confused signals and will be unable to generate success and stability in the interview. Likewise, if you instruct your body to be healthy while feeling angry or sad, you are most likely to throw a spanner in the works and produce a poor or low quality outcome.

So while meditating use lots of positive visualisations, bright life affirming and spiritual images and mood enhancing words. You can take a word like happy and while repeating it in your mind, think of the feelings you get when you are happy. You will find by repeating this word you will induce this state in the body. The next time you are in a negative situation, you can say this word in your mind, and the association in your subconscious if it has been implanted repeatedly, will immediately start to cause changes in the body to recreate these feelings and then change your mood.

You can apply different words in your meditations to induce different states of mind. Such as happy, relax, release, health, strength, power, peace and love etc. Just repeat these positive images and feelings into your subconscious and you will eventually find that you are creating a permanent state of positive well being and health there, the subconscious will then recreate the same in your body.

Outside of Qi Gong practice, you can also create positive affirmations for your mind by surrounding it with symbolism that promotes love, happiness, and tranquillity. Everything from positive religious statues to soothing colours to lucky charms and talisman. All of them will have a subtle and influential impact on the health of your mind and body. If you imagine being in a room with a smiling Buddha statue, you are obviously less likely to feel angry and so forth. So ensure for your good health to surround yourself with positive imagery.

You can even write positive messages on sticky pads in key areas around your home, car or work place. When seeing these affirmations they will refocus and inspire your mind towards its goals.

Be aware, that if you do the opposite and surround your self with dark, violent, sad or oppressive imagery or music, then that is what your subconscious will focus on and try to generate in your actual life. This will not bring you the happiness you desire, but will instead ultimately lead you towards more suffering and pain. So be cautious in the choices of what you are allowing around you and encouraging into your mind.

This also includes many of the soap operas and programs that we now watch on TV, or films we view in the cinema. These are being viewed by two minds in you, the conscious which is seeing them just as entertainment and the subconscious which sees them more so as instructive. When they are portraying negativity, such as gossiping, arguing, betrayal, despair, hatred and so forth. Then all of that is being absorbed but not logically filtered by the subconscious, which will in turn try to recreate events in your life to bring them or similar experiences to you. Just like the way the subconscious will bring you the red balloon even if you don't want it, as we discussed earlier in the book. So be very careful what you watch and invite into your mind.

Now back to the routine…

Step 3) The Inner Smile.

Create a real smile on your face, filling it with warmth, love, peace and happiness. Then imagine that this smile is drifting down the front of your body. Melting through the muscles, filling them with joy and affection. Repeat this again, sending the smile down through the centre of the body, spreading warmth and love through the organs. And finally once more, down the back of your body.

4) Bathing In The Sun.

Bring the conscious thought up into your head and focus it on the area between your eyebrows. Now imagine the area filling with the warming and glowing golden light of the sun. This energy is empowering and refreshing you. Feel it spread throughout your whole body as if you are standing, bathed in the glorious rays of heat and light from the sun on a hot summers day. Absorb its energy and power.

5) Filling With Power.

Breathe deeply right down to your lower belly, beneath the navel, down to the lower dantian. Fill this area with energy. Concentrate the minds focus to this point. Wherever you concentrate your intent on, your energy will flow to. Now imagine a glowing ball of vibrant bright shining energy. As you inhale, it expands and grows larger, as you exhale you contract and condense this powerful energy. Imagine this ball is full of raw power and electricity and is now providing your kidneys and digestion with great power to help them function better.

After eight breaths, begin again, but this time grow the energy in the centre of your chest, the middle dantian. Fill this ball with energy, peace, calmness, compassion and love.

After another four breaths, create a new ball of energy in your mind between the eyebrows, in the upper dantian. Fill this area with energy, intelligence, wisdom and understanding. After four more breaths move on to the next step.

6) Connecting To The Higher Source.

In this part of the meditation, connect to your God. Whether that is God, Spirit, Universe or some form of higher energy and intelligence, then that is up to you. But feel its love and acceptance and feel gratitude for it. Take a few moments to connect and pray deeply for love, happiness and wisdom in your life.

7) Positive Affirmations.

Your subconscious mind should have become quieter by now and should be in a more suggestible and easily influenced state. So take advantage of this and start to implant suggestions into it of who you want to become. Remember to focus on what you want to be rather than on what you want to get rid of, as often the subconscious is prone to try to create whatever you are thinking of, be it in your interests or not. So always focus clearly on and attach good emotions and feelings to what you want to achieve.

You can make up whatever affirmations you choose, just be sure to make them meaningful and productive for your life. You can say things such as "with every breath I take, I am filled with an abundance of peace and love". Or if you had a weak heart, you could say "Everyday my heart is becoming incredibly powerful and strong". Or if you had trouble sleeping, "Every night I will go to bed and get to sleep easily and quickly. I will sleep deeply and soundly, and arise feeling refreshed and revived in the morning".

When you say your affirmations, be sure to attach a good positive upbeat feeling to them. You may also want to repeat the most important ones several times over in your head.

8) Stillness And Quiet.

For the last part of the meditation, you should try to turn the mind completely off or at least minimize it down to as few thoughts as you can.

It is very normal for thoughts and distractions to keep popping up from the subconscious mind. There are many methods used to try to reduce these …

You can become the observer, and just watch the thought as it comes up into the mind and then moves through it and out of it. Don't become involved or interfere with it. Just observe it.

Or another method is to give your thoughts a quick answer, yes or no, or later for any complicated thoughts. This tends to be quite effective and should halt the same questions from repeating on you.

You could also engage the conscious mind to focus on just one action. This strengthens the conscious mind and pulls energy and power away from the subconscious. You can focus on your breathing or on a spot in your visual field or even on a candle. Focusing the mind on simply following the inhale and exhale of your breath is probably the most common and widely used method to quiet the mind during meditation.

Whatever you do, don't try too hard to fight or suppress the thoughts. By doing this you are in fact feeding them and will most likely encourage more of them. Instead be calm, relax, tell your subconscious that it is being turned off and then just flow with whatever happens. Some days are good and quiet, other days are not. But eventually over time, and it may take a long time, even years of practice, you will eventually find your subconscious quietens and your body, energy, mind and spirit become much stronger in all aspects of health and happiness. After several minutes in this meditation, gently come out of it and carry on with your day.

How much time you spend in Qi Gong is up to you. Most people need to do at least 10 to 15 minutes daily to derive any benefit from it. A good and highly productive routine would be 25 to 40 minutes daily.

Qi Gong is working on long term principles of accumulating small amounts of energy over time, eventually leading to a big reserve of it in your body.

Positive mental and emotional changes will only occur through repeated efforts of reprogramming your subconscious.

So don't expect overnight results from Qi Gong, Yoga or meditation. Instead be prepared for long term effort leading gradually to much higher standards of well being and health in all aspects of your life.

Personally I have found Qi Gong to be one of the most rewarding and beneficial activities you could possibly do. Initially it does take time and effort from you, but long term it will reward your small daily investment with a magnificent return.

Chapter Seventy Nine   -   The Pillars Of Health.

As we are approaching the end of the book, it is now time to revise and summarize some of the many new and different methods we have learnt from the Eastern ways of health.

However, before we do that we need to learn something very important about how the subconscious mind works in many of us. Be aware that for most people, although we might like to think that we are open minded and are giving everything a fair and true hearing, our subconscious minds may not be so, indeed they may have a very different agenda. The subconscious and the ego that resides within it, prefers always to be right, it certainly does not want to hear anything that is unfamiliar and a challenge to its preformed beliefs. It has invested much time and effort in these ideas, and they now even underpin its existence.

Its immediate reaction in many people is to nearly always defend these memorized ideas against anything new and different. It does this sometimes by simply ignoring the immediate facts, truth and logic presented to it. Often by trying to exaggerate and over value anything that sounds familiar to its own beliefs, and at the same time playing down and diminishing anything that goes against these ideas. So you must be watchful of this, as the conscious and subconscious may not be following the same path. Indeed the subconscious can play many games with us and close our minds to truth and awareness, leading us to much illness, pain and unnecessary suffering in our lives.

As we have grown up in the West our subconscious has been blasted with the authority and self proclaimed supremacy of Western Medicine, many of us invested our faith strongly in it simply because there didn't seem to be any other viable alternative. We have become somewhat brainwashed by this and have closed our minds to thinking rationally and judging things in a fair way. This is why so many people do not question their Western doctors about the validity and even success rate of any proposed treatment, but instead often just blindly follow whatever they are told to do.

Because of this it will be difficult for some people to open their minds enough to start to reassess the credibility of thoughts that have been placed into their subconscious.

The first step to resolving this dilemma is to become aware that this is how your subconscious is behaving. By being aware of it, it will weaken its ability to continue damaging us in this negative frame of mind. It will even start to riddle its foundations with doubt, which should eventually lead to a clear reassessment of the so called facts that it had established within it.

Secondly, in reference to this book if we have opened our conscious minds and accepted these new ideas as being logical and truthful then by reading and rereading the chapters from this book it will start to push them into your subconscious and they will eventually become part of you, putting you back in charge and allowing you to take control of your health and your happiness. Whether that is through Chinese Medicine or a more judgemental and clear headed view of what is really effective or perhaps not so good in Western Medicine.

I recommend that you read this book at least once every six months for the next couple of years to allow your subconscious to become accustomed to and adopt this fresh perspective of your health through the theories and philosophies of Eastern Medicines. If you do this, it will allow this great knowledge to sink deeply into your mind, alter your perspectives and start you on the path to a freer, healthier and more joyful existence.

The Pillars.

1) Balance.

One of the biggest ideas we need to incorporate into our lives is the wisdom of balance. To balance Yin with Yang, hot with cold, activity with rest and so forth.

When we find ourselves pushed to any extreme then we can easily damage our bodies and create illness in them. If we also stay too long on one side or the other then this too can weaken us and lead to sickness. So we must always strive to balance our internal and external conditions to keep us in the middle where everything is strong and running at peak levels. To put it simply, if you find yourself too hot then do or take something that cools you down, if you are overworked then rest up, if you have rested too long then get active and so on.

Once you become aware and watchful then your subconscious will eventually take notice and automatically start to guide you back to where it is healthy and productive in the middle.

2) The Big Picture.

Always look at the condition in terms of the big picture and not just the little ones. When you are treating an illness or trying to make yourself more healthy, always look at every aspect of your life, your emotions, your environment, your physical activity or lack thereof, your sleep, your work, your social life and so forth. Everything is interconnected and vital, nothing can be left out or ignored. When you change one, it will impact on the others. So you need to respect all areas, the mind, the body and the spirit. There is no point in having a muscular or toned body at the expense of the spirit and mind or vice versa.

By keeping this general bigger view of everything in balance, then it tends to bring all the smaller pictures into alignment and everything flourishes.

3) Power Up Your Qi.

Keep your energy strong and maintained at as high levels as you possibly can. There is nothing in the body or outside of it for that matter that does not utilize energy to function. If your energy is weak, then the mind, spirit and the body will all begin to function at a lower rate. This can lead to ailments or at the very least reduce your standard of living.

So keep your energy charged up, empowering you and your body to run at the highest levels of performance. Deep breathing, Qi Gong and white rice are all excellent providers of good beneficial energy in the body.

4) Nourish Your Blood And Nutrients.

Along with the Qi, the other side of the body is your nutrients. The energy takes these more physical blocks and uses them to construct a vessel for your spirit. If you do not eat properly and provide your system with wholesome nourishing foods then you cannot expect your body to be maintained and rebuilt into a healthy form.

5) Preserve Your Jing.

Your Jing essence creates your hormones which keep you strong, healthy, vibrant and young. When they begin to run out you start to age and weaken. The more excessive our lifestyles, the more we will live off of our adrenalin and other hormones. The more we overwork, over exercise, stress ourselves and generally do too much, then the quicker we will use up our Jing, speed up the rate at which we age and even shorten our lifespan on this earth. So slow down, take things more moderately and don't burn yourself out.

6) Diet.

There are many suggestions to follow for a healthy way of eating, so we will just list the main ones here …

Balance your foods. Eat according to the internal and external conditions you find yourself in. When you are cold eat warming foods, when you are hot eat cooling ones and so forth.

The five flavours generally indicate how a food will behave inside our bodies.

The bitter taste generally cools and detoxifies. However too much of it can dry you out and deplete your system of energy and nutrients.

The sweet taste nourishes and builds energy when it is consumed in small amounts, but it can block you up, make you toxic and over heat you in large ones.

The spicy pungent aromatic flavour moves, expectorates, activates and warms. But too much of it can over heat you, burn up your energy and nutrients, and then tire you out.

The salty flavour moves, moistens, cools, astringes and breaks up lumps. If you have too much of it, it can steal your energy and make things slow excessively, leading to cold and dampness on the inside.

The sour taste can tighten and hold things in, which can help build up levels of nutrients, blood and hormones in the body. But too much of it can over tighten, strangle and seize you up.

The mouth often lets us feel and know what general reaction a food is going to have in the rest of the body. Heat generating stimulants like alcohol and spices can feel like they are enlivening, activating and burning. Whereas damp producing foods like bananas can leave the mouth sticky and gooey. And bitter purging foods like pomegranates can leave them feeling dry.

The main heating foods are coffee, alcohol, spices, chocolate and dark teas. These are all stimulants, you only need a small amount of them in your diet to have a big impact inside of you. It is easy to understand this if you think of the effect of petrol being poured on to a fire, a small amount can create a very big and powerful reaction. Sugars and fats will also generate heat in the body, but unlike the others they will start to glue it up as well.

The main cooling foods are fruits, vegetables and beans. Remember to add energy producing white rice and small amounts of spice to your vegetables to give your digestion power to break them down and absorb the heavier and cooler particles from them.

The main drying foods are bitter fruit and juices which cool and dry. And alcohol, spices and coffee which heat and dry.

The main damp forming foods are oils, dairy, bananas, sweet fruits, sugars and fats.

To make the most of the natural power that moves through your digestion have a big breakfast, medium lunch and small dinner. This will help you better digest your food, give you more energy, power up your organs and keep your weight at a more correct level.

To keep your digestive tract healthy, wash and clean it between meals with green and peppermint teas and bitter juice such as pomegranate, grape and berries.

Try to always have hot food or at least a hot drink with your meals. This helps your stomach to break down foods and saves energy for it and the rest of your body.

Cravings are often telling us that we are missing some form of nutrient from within our system. If you are getting them, then try adding densely nutritious foods like plant oils, nuts, seeds and eggs into your diet. Also add in plenty of white rice if you are getting sugar or other stimulant cravings, as these indicate your energy levels are too low.

Try to avoid consuming processed foods and instead try to eat natural and organic foods whenever you can. These foods are less toxic and the body is designed to break them down more easily.

Avoid dairy and animal fats. They will block you up and create phlegm and toxins which will increase your risks of many serious diseases.

The main wholesome energy producing food is white rice. But if your system has cooled down too much, then for a quick pick me up you can use small amounts of alcohol, coffee and spices to rev things up and get them going again.

Don't overfill your stomach. Eat only until you are about four fifths full. This will leave room for your stomach to work on breaking down the meal and adding digestive juices to it.

If you are hot and stressed have lots of cooling, moving and relaxing peppermint tea.

7) Breathe Deeply.

Breathing is our primary source of energy. When we breathe properly we fill ourselves with power and we also help to expel toxins and waste from our blood stream and bodies. We should perform abdominal breathing throughout our day and emphasize complete breathing when we are exercising and meditating.

If we are feeling tired during the day, it is quite beneficial to take a break and perform deep breathing exercises for two minutes. This will flush our minds and bodies with oxygen and energy, and get us alert and going again.

8) Maintain Good Posture.

To facilitate our breathing we should stand or sit in a comfortably erect position. This allows our lungs and all other organs to operate more freely and effectively. And also influences our subconscious to adopt and keep a more positive mental outlook.

9) Wrap Up Well.

Respect the weather and protect yourself from over exposure to heat, cold, rain, wind and dryness. The elements can quickly deplete you of energy and nutrients or can lodge in your system causing it to become damaged. So simply wear the right clothes to balance and protect yourself against the elements, and avoid over exposure to any extremes or for excessively long periods.

10) Follow The Seasons.

Again look at the big picture. See the Winter as a time to slow down, recuperate and build up nutrients and reserves in your body. See the Summer as a time to become more active and alive again. This is just like the way we see every other living being in this world respond to the seasons and the natural cycles of the earth. We have all evolved and are programmed to fit in with these rhythms, and by doing so it helps to keep us in a healthy state of balance.

11) Sleep Well.

Get to bed before 11pm if you want to stay young and refreshed. This will maximize your bodies release of regenerating hormones. We need good sleep to rest ourselves and to replenish our Yin after the Yang activities of the day. We also need to turn our conscious minds off or else they may become overloaded and lead us towards mental disorder, or even madness and breakdown.

12) Exercise The Middle Way.

If we do too little, then everything begins to lodge and stagnate within us and are unused and neglected muscles will begin to sag and weaken. If we do too much we use and burn up our blood, energy, nutrients and hormones and we wear out our joints and other parts. So we should do neither, not too much nor too little, but instead a more moderate and frequent amount of exercise. This will invigorate and encourage circulation through our systems without wearing things out, damaging them or using them up.

13) Sex.

If we are male we can make too many demands on our Jing essence and hormones by having sex too frequently. So as we age or if we are in poor health we should have sex less often. Or alternately we can adopt Tantric or Taoist style sexual techniques and continue to have plenty of it, but refrain from the physical act of ejaculation every single time we have sex. These methods will also enhance our sex lives, making the experience more pleasurable for both ourselves and our partners.

All the next pillars concern the mind and the spirit ...

14) Positivity Versus Negativity.

Choose to think happy. Always look on the bright side of things and fill your mind with as much genuine love and happiness as you can. These are the only emotions that not just make you feel alive and make you want to live but also bring health to your body. All the other negative emotions will weaken you and eventually cause disease in your system and suffering in your mind and soul.

15) Fix Your Organs To Fix Your Mind.

If you want a healthy and happy mind then take care of your organs, as they are feeding your brain with energy, nutrients and hormones. If you let the physical side of you weaken, then less good stuff gets up to support your mind and your mood and mental functioning will falter and start to drop.

16) Be Careful What You Let In.

Don't feed your mind negativity. Whether that is people, books, movies, TV programs or some other form of media. If you want happiness then you must practice living it. So constantly try to reinforce positive messages into your subconscious and steer clear of any negative influences.

17) Master Your Emotions.

Think deeply about each emotion and become aware of how they behave in your body, then question their existence. Should they be in you, are they helping you or harming you, do you really want many of them, do you really want emotions like anger or fear interfering with or even destroying your life ? If you don't, then start to let them go. Become the observer, watch them as they arise in your mind but don't let them take control of it. Instead reject them and tell them you don't want them in your life anymore. Keep repeating this message to them and into your subconscious until they weaken and fade away. It may take many months or even years of practice but eventually the time will come when you will be fully in charge of your mind again.

When you have changed your beliefs about emotions, you will find that this changes the emotions attached to your past memories. It diminishes the destructive elements joined to negative memories that have kept your mind imprisoned, but leaves the wisdom and lessons learnt from whatever bad experiences you have had so you can make better decisions when dealing with others in your future.

18) Free Yourself From Society.

Don't blindly follow others. Stop having faith in people with empty promises. If they have repeatedly let you down and given you bad advice, then don't be foolish, don't keep following them. No matter what new hype, propaganda and shiny dazzling lies they are now peddling, break free from this and from allowing them to control, manipulate and mislead you. Be they politicians, celebrities, governments, TV producers, capitalists, religious leaders or any others who have put themselves into positions of power or authority.

This world is about you and God, no one else owns you, don't be conned or bullied into giving your freedom away. Instead open your mind and use it. Question everything and think for yourself. Think deeply and come to your own conclusions about what will bring meaning, fulfilment and happiness to your own life. It's your life, don't let anyone else abuse you and tell you how you must live and fit into their rules, and then stop you from having your freedom and the joy that you are entitled to.

19) Lose The Fight.

When possible stop fighting events and people who are in your way. It is often far easier to approach your destination from a different angle. You don't have to climb over every mountain, it is much simpler just to walk around them. You will find that most of the time you will achieve much more through a calm, clear and logical approach, than through an aggressive one. It is obviously far healthier for the body to live this way too.

20) Practice Qi Gong And Meditation.

Apart from all the physical and energetic benefits, Qi Gong and meditation are one of the best ways to empower and free your mind. The quiet and focusing techniques strengthen your conscious mind and in the process also weaken the chattering monkey and ego of the subconscious. Thus bringing you health, clarity, power and joy.

21) Do Good.

Quite simply, when you project real love and goodness from your being you are bringing your mind into a state of positivity which is immediately rewarding you with health, peace, meaning and happiness.

Whereas when you do wrong your mind is now in a negative state which can only further rot your subconscious and lead to illness within the mind and body.

Further problems often ensue from the fruition of any negative seeds you have planted around you. Or in other words, the more people you annoy the higher the likelihood of eventually meeting someone who causes you a lot of serious problems.

22) Live Through Your Soul.

Temporary pleasurable highs can be found in your ego, but with these they will always eventually be accompanied by a downside. Instead if you invest in your soul, you will experience a new sense of love, joy, contentment and happiness that cannot be found through any other means.

On top of this the soul is the only eternal creation in this world. You cannot take your ego, your wealth, your cars, your status, your property or anything else with you when you pass over. So if you have neglected and not empowered your real self, your soul, then you will truly have very little in the next world.

Chapter Eighty - Your Health Is In Your Hands.

For many of us life has never been easy, but it now seems to be getting harder and harder to stay physically and emotionally healthy in our modern world. The incidence of most illnesses are escalating dramatically. Every part of us seems to be under more general threat than ever before. Our physical bodies from an ever increasing number of pollutants and chemicals in our environment. And also from poor quality and modified unnatural foods. Our minds too are battered from junk TV and from our hectic fast paced and information overloaded lifestyles. And our spirits from the corruption, greed, negativity and moral vacuity which seems to have seeped into all aspects of structured society around us. From big businesses intent on taking over the world, to the propaganda of dirty politics, to cheap mindless and often degrading and demoralising entertainment. Life does seem to be becoming more and more difficult. Even the rich and famous cannot seem to escape illness in both their bodies and minds, they too, just like the rest of us, are affected and plagued by the emptiness and pollution of our modern apathetic uncaring society.

So the question has become, how do we fix this ? How do we get out of this mess ? How do we survive this onslaught and make ourselves healthy ? Well it would be great if there was a magic pill we all could take, or even better a magic wand we could wave to cure all illnesses and change everything for the better. But just like other fairy tales, magic pills don't exist in real life and they never will.

However, even though we are surrounded by more negative forces than ever before, if we are patient and we practice and work steadily, then through the principles of Eastern Medicines and philosophies, we will find ourselves becoming more healthy than we ever thought possible. With these methods we can empower and free ourselves, and every single aspect of us can change for the better. We can maintain, strengthen, heal, protect, enhance and regenerate our bodies more efficiently and effectively. We can control and master our emotions, instead of them controlling and manipulating us. We can bring clarity, peace, intelligence and wisdom to our minds. And we can start to bring our souls and all the real joy and love contained within them out into our lives and the world around us.

It will take time and effort, but if you are willing to properly follow the ways of the East, you will be rewarded in abundance for the work you have put into it. In particular if you continue the path of spiritual attainment, pushing the mind and soul to higher levels, you will find true enlightenment and a priceless prize at the end of the journey.

With this book you have been given an opportunity for a fresh start to enhance your life, you have been presented with a wealth of information which can help guide you on this beautiful and wonderful journey towards great health and real happiness in your body, mind and spirit.

The famous Chinese philosopher Lao Tzu once said, "*A journey of a thousand miles begins with a single step*". So decide today that it is time to take this step and to make the change for a new way, a new life, a new brighter future, where you will walk hand in hand with your wisdom, your freedom, your soul, your health and your happiness.

You now have the knowledge to begin to create superior health, wisdom and love. All you need is a just a little time, patience and perseverance. If you can give just this much, you will eventually succeed.

"Our greatest glory is not in never falling, but in rising every time we fall."

- Confucius

~~~~~~~~~~

~~~

For further resources and information on general health and well being, and on Eastern Medicines and philosophies, please check out our website

www.superiorhealthawaitsyou.com

Or

www.myleswray.com

You will find interesting frequently updated articles and other resources available there.

And also a collection of downloadable Qi Gong training clips and other health enhancing media.

References And Sources.   -   All Internet Sites Accessed June 2010.

---------------------------------- Introduction ----------------------------------

- World Alzheimer's Report -
http://www.alz.co.uk/research/files/WorldAlzheimerReport-ExecutiveSummary.pdf
- Martin Knapp, The London School Of Economics,
Martin Prince, Institute Of Psychiatry, Kings College London -
http://www2.lse.ac.uk/newsAndMedia/news/archives/2007/AlzheimersReport.aspx
- Access Economics, Keeping Dementia Front Of Mind: Incidence And Prevalence 2009 - 2050, commissioned by Alzheimer's Australia. www.alzheimers.org.au/content.cfm?infopageid=6012
- The Alzheimer's Society of Scotland report - The Dementia Epidemic.
http://www.alzscot.org/pages/media/dementia_epidemic.htm
- Messerli F. et al, Hypertension : uncontrolled and conquering the world, The Lancet ;370(9587): 539, 18-08-07.
- Premature births - Behrman R. et al, National Academy of Sciences Institute Of Medicine, 2007.
- Official figures on cancer obtained from parliamentary questions by the Liberal Democrats in '09
http://www.libdems.org.uk/press_releases_detail.aspx?title=Cancers_related_to_alcohol_consumption_up_50%25_says_Foster_&pPK=1c402b3b-f3dd-4a2b-ae3a-fa9985eb7c13
- Bowel cancer figures '09 - www.beatingbowelcancer.org/Resources/Downloads/PR%20090331.pdf
- Boyle P., Levin B., World Cancer Report 2008, IARC Nonserial Publication, World Health Org.
- Teresa E. Seeman et al, Disability trends among older Americans, AJPH, Jan 2010, Vol. 100, No 1.
- Carlos Blanco et al, Mental health of college students and their non college attending peers, Arch Gen Psychiatry,2008,65(12):1429-1437
- Diagnosed Attention Deficit Hyperactivity Disorder and Learning Disability : United States, 2004-2006, Vital And Health Statistics, July 2008, Series 10, No. 237.
- Australian Bureau of Statistics - Mental health
http://www.abs.gov.au/AUSSTATS/abs@.nsf/Lookup/4102.0Main+Features30March%202009
- National Statistics, The health of children and young people.
http://www.statistics.gov.uk/children/downloads/mental_health.pdf
- Sylvana Cote et al, Depression and anxiety symptoms : onset, developmental course and risk factors during early childhood, J. Child Psychol. and Psych., Vol. 50 is.10, p 1201-1208, online 10 Jun '09.
- E L Masso Gonzalez et al, Trends in the prevalence and incidence of diabetes in the UK, J Epidemiol Community Health 2009;63:332-336.
- Green F, Ryan C, An overview of chronic kidney disease in Australia, 27 May 2009, Australian Institute of Health and Welfare.
- Skin Cancer, Scotland. http://info.cancerresearchuk.org/news/archive/cancernews/2009-04-29-figures-published-on-cancer-rates-in-scotland
- Foresight, Tackling obesities - future choices. http://www.foresight.gov.uk/obesity/20.pdf
- Wang Y. et al, Will all Americans become overweight or obese? Estimating the progression and cost of the US obesity epidemic, Obesity 2008;16(1):2323-2330.
- Simpson CR et al, Trends in the epidemiology and prescribing of medication for eczema in England, Journal of the Royal Society of Medicine 2009, 102(3):108- 17.

---------------------------------- Chapter 10 ----------------------------------

- Tsunehara C. et al, Diet of second generation Japanese-American men with and without non insulin-dependant diabetes, Am. J. Clin. Nutri. 52(1990):731-738.
- Murgatroyd C., Dynamic DNA Methylation persistent adverse effects of early life stress, Nature Neuroscience 13, 649(2010) .
- DNA damage caused by pesticides, David Loyn, BBC News, 19-05-08. / S. Kaur, Patiala University. http://news.bbc.co.uk/2/hi/7407707.stm
- Dean Ornish et al, Changes in prostate gene expression in men undergoing an intensive nutrition and lifestyle intervention. PNAS,2008, 105(24),8369-8374.
- Feeling car sick, B. Goldsmith for Reuters. http://www.reuters.com/article/idUSSP16191020080915 / Hilton A. et al, Aston University.

---------------------------------- Chapter 26 ----------------------------------

- Eigenmann P., Haenggeli C., Food colourings, preservatives and hyperactivity, The Lancet, Vol. 370 Is. 9598, Nov 2007. P1524-1525.
- McCann D. et al, Food additives and hyperactive behaviour, The Lancet Nov 07; 370(9598): 1560-7.
- Akbaraly T. et al, Dietary pattern and depressive symptoms in middle age, British Journal Of Psychiatry, 2009,195:408-413.

- Pierce D. et al, Over eating by young obesity prone and lean rats caused by tastes associated with low energy foods, Obesity 2007;15:1969-1979.
- Swithers S., Davidson T., A role for sweet taste: Calorie predictive relations in energy regulation by rats, Behavioral Neuroscience Feb 2008;122(1).
- Fry ups raise bowel cancer risk, BBC , 26-08-08. http://news.bbc.co.uk/2/hi/health/7581916.stm / World Cancer Research Fund
- Nothlings U. et al, Meat and fat intake as risks for pancreatic cancer : the multiethnic cohort study, J National Cancer Inst 2005;97(19):1458-65.
- Larsson S. et al, Processed meat consumption, dietary nitrosamines and stomach cancer risk in a cohort of Swedish women, Int J Cancer Aug 2006; 119(4):915-9.
- Pereira M. et al, Breakfast eating and weight change in a five year prospective of adolescents: project eat (eating among teens), Pediatrics March 2008; 121(3):638-645.
- Arble D. et al, Circadian timing of food intake contribute to weight gain, Obesity '09, 17 11,2100-2.
- Jakubowicz D., Virginia Commonwealth University, Big breakfast helped women lose weight, study presented to Endocrine's Society 90th Annual Meeting, San Francisco 17-06-08.
- Pereira M. et al, Breakfast eating and weight change, Paediatrics, 2008;121, e638-e645.
--------------------------------- Chapter 28 ---------------------------------
- Key T. et al, Cancer incidence in British vegetarians, Br. Journal of Cancer (2009), 101, 192-197.
- Chan J. et al, Vegetable and fruit intake and pancreatic cancer, Canc. Epid. Biom. and Prev., Sep 2005, 14; 2093.
- Rosen E. et al, BRCA1 and BRCA2 as molecular targets for phytochemicals, Brit. J. Of Cancer, (2006) 94, 407-426.
- World Hunger hits one billion, BBC News, 19-06-09. UN Food and Agriculture Organisation 2009. http://news.bbc.co.uk/2/hi/europe/8109698.stm
- Min Zhang, Dietary intakes of mushrooms and green tea combine to reduce the risk of breast cancer, Int. J. Of Cancer, V 124 Is 6, 1404-1408, 01-10-08.
- Kulczyski et al, Milk and colic, Acta Paediatr., Washington University School of Medicine, 2000.
- Chan J. et al, Dairy products and calcium risk in Physicians Health Study, Am. J. Of Clin. Nutrition, 74 : 549-554, Oct 2001.
- Breast cancer and milk intake, Milksucks.com, http://www.milksucks.com/breast.asp
- Segall J. et al, Dietary lactose as a possible risk factor for ischemic heart disease, Int. J. Of Cardiology, 46, 3 (1994), 197-207.
- Osteoporosis and milk intake, Milksucks.com, http://www.milksucks.com/osteo.asp
- Nsouli T. et al, Role of food allergy in serious otitis media, Ann. Allergy Asthma Immunol., 1995 Mar;74(3);277-8.
- Larsson S. et al, Milk and lactose intakes and ovarian cancer risk, Am. J. Of Clin. Nutr., V80,No5,1353-1357, Nov 2004.
- Ghosh D. et al, Effects of anthocyanins and other phenolic of boysenberry and blackcurrant as inhibitors of oxidative stress and damage..., J. of Sc. Food and Agri., V86 Is5, p678-686, 23-01-2006.
- Kurowska E., Citrus peel can lower cholesterol, J. Agriculture And Food Chemistry, 12-05-04.
- Blueberries lower cholesterol, BBC News, 24-08-04. http://news.bbc.co.uk/2/hi/health/3591384.stm Agnes Rimando et al, US department of Agriculture.
- Dai Q. et al, Fruit and vegetable juice and Alzheimer's' disease, Am. J. Med. '06 Sep. 119(9):751-9.
- Gordillo G. et al, Oral administration of blueberry inhibits angiogenic tumour growth, Antioxidants and Redox Sig., 01-01-2009, V 11(1), 47-58.
- Stoner G. et al, Anthocyanins in black raspberries prevent oesophageal tumors in rats, Cancer Prevention Research 2009 2;84
- Ray R. et al, Bitter melon extract inhibits breast cancer cell prolif., Can. Res., 01-03-10, 70;1925.
- Seymour E. et al, Chronic intake of phytochemical enriched diet ..., J Gerontol A Biol Sci Med Sci (2008) 63 (10) :1034-1042.
- Spencer J. et al, Blueberry induced changes in spatial working memory ..., Free Radical Biology and Medicine Aug 2008; 45(3):295-305
- Pomegranates fruity panacea, BBC News, 28-11-04. M. Aviram et al, Rambam Medical Centre. http://news.bbc.co.uk/2/hi/health/3937053.stm
- Pantuck A. et al, Phase ii study of pomegranate juice ..., Clin. Cancer Research, July 06, 12; 4018.
- Xianglin Shi, Grape seed extract kills laboratory leukaemia cells, Clin. Cancer Research, 01-01-09.
- Ford A. et al, Effect of fibre, antispasmodics and peppermint oil in the treatment of irritable bowel syndrome,BMJ2008;337:a2313.
- Gasiewicz T. et al, Identification of potential aryl hydrocarbon receptor antagonists in green tea, Chemical Research in Toxicology 2003; 16(7):865-872.
- Jun Tan et al, Green Tea Epigallocatechin-3-gallate..., J Neurosci, 21-09-05, 25 (38) ; 8807-8814.
- Cardelli J. et al, Tea Polyphenols decrease serum levels of prostate specific antigen ..., 1940-6207.CAPR-08-0167v1.
- Wu Ah et al, Green tea and risk of breast cancer in Asian Americans, Int. J. Of Cancer 2003;106(4):574-9.
- Setiawan V. et al, Protective effect of green tea on the risk of chronic gastritis and stomach cancer, Int. J. Of Cancer

2001;92(2):600-4.
- Tokunaga S. et al, Green tea consumption and serum lipids…, Ann. of Epidim. 2002;12(3):157-65.
- Sinha R. et al, Meat intake and mortality, Arch Intern Med,V169,No6, March 23 2009.
- Chong E. et al, Red meat and chicken consumption …, Am. J. of Epidem., 2009;169(7):867-76.
- Taylor E. et al, Meat consumption and risk of breast cancer in the UK, Br J Cancer, 2007 April 10; 96(7):1139-1146.
- Stolzenberg-Solomon R. et al, Dietary fatty acids and pancreatic cancer in the NIH-AARP diet and health study, J Nat Cancer Ins 2009; 101(14):1001-1011.
---------------------------------- Chapter 32 ----------------------------------
- Lange P. et al, Developing COPD: a 25 year follow up study of the general population, Thorax 2006;61:935-939.
- Alonso A. et al, Risk of dementia hospitalisation associated with cardiovascular risk factors in mid life and old age, J Neurol Neurosurg Psychiatry 2009;80:1194-1201.
---------------------------------- Chapter 36 ----------------------------------
- Is your desk making you sick, D. Williams CNN, Charles Gerba University of Arizona. www.cnn.com/2004/HEALTH/12/13/cold.flu.desk/index.html
- MRSA super bug found in ocean and public beaches, S. Sternberg, USA Today, 12-09-2009, http://www.usatoday.com/news/health/2009-09-12-staph-superbug-MRSA-beaches_N.htm
Roberts M. et al, University of Washington.
- Faecal bacteria join the commute, BBC News, 15-10-08, http://news.bbc.co.uk/2/hi/7667499.stm
Curtis V. et al, London School of Hygiene and Tropical Medicine.
- Mothers were right over colds, BBC, 14-11-05. Eccles R., Common Cold Centre, Cardiff University. http://news.bbc.co.uk/2/hi/uk_news/wales/4433496.stm
- Gardner E., Ritz B., Malnutrition and energy restriction differentially affect viral immunity, J. Nutr. 136,1141-1144, may 2006.
---------------------------------- Chapter 37 ----------------------------------
- Cancer cases at all time high, BBC, 07-01-04, UK Association of Cancer Registries. http://news.bbc.co.uk/2/hi/health/3373447.stm
- Stattin P. et al, Prospective study of hypoglycaemia and cancer risk, Diabetes Care March 2007;30(3):561-567.
- Bunin G. et al, A case control study of childhood brain tumours and fathers hobbies, CCC 2008;19(10):1201-7.
- Malekzadeh R. et al, Tea drinking habits and oesophageal cancer, BMJ 2009;338:b929.
---------------------------------- Chapter 39 ----------------------------------
- Dobnig H. et al, Independent association of low serum 25-hydroxyvitamin d and 1,25-dihydroxyvit d levels with all cause and cardiovascular mortality, Arch Intern Med 2008;168(12):1246.
- Parker J. et al, Levels of vitamin D and cardiometabolic disorders reviews, Maturitas, March 2010;65(3):225-236.
---------------------------------- Chapter 40 ----------------------------------
- Hansen J., Light at night, shift work and breast cancer risk, J Nat. Canc. Inst. 2001,93(20):1513-5.
---------------------------------- Chapter 41 ----------------------------------
- Too little sleep may make you fat, BBC, 22-11-04, http://news.bbc.co.uk/2/hi/health/4026133.stm
Gangwisch J. et al, Columbia University.
---------------------------------- Chapter 42 ----------------------------------
- Wojnar M. et al, Sleep problems and suicidality in the national co morbidity survey replication, J Psychiatric Research 2009;43(5):526-31.
- Cohen S. et al, Sleep habits and susceptibility to the common cold, Arch Int Med 2009;169(1):62-67
- Knutson K. et al, Association between sleep and blood pressure in mid life, Arch Intern Med 2009; 169(11):1055-61.
- Vgontzas A. et al, Insomnia with objective short sleep duration is associated with high risk for hypertensio, Sleep;32(04):491-497.
- Gangwisch, Sleep and teen depression, Columbia University Medical centre, presented to Sleep 2009, Seattle, Associated Professional Sleep Societies.
- Kazuo Eguchi et al, Short sleep duration as independent indicator of cardiovascular events … , Arch Intern Med 2008; 168(20):2225-2231
- Ayas N. et al, A prospective study of sleep duration and coronary heart disease in women, Arch Intern Med 2003;163:205-209.
- Kakizaki M. et al, Sleep duration and risk of breast cancer 08 Nov 4; 99(9):1502-05.
---------------------------------- Chapter 46 ----------------------------------
- Caution killing germs may be hazardous to your health, J. Adler, J. Interlandi, Newsweek, 20-10-07. www.newsweek.com/2007/10/20/caution-killing-germs-may-be-hazardous-to-your-health.html
- Sudden Cardiac Death: Should young athletes be screened, E. Harrell, Time, 10-09-09. Int Olympic Committee. www.time.com/time/health/article/0,8599,1921260,00.html
- Hidden heart problems for college athletes, A. Grayson, ABC news 30-03-09.

www.abcnews.go.com/Health/HeartDiseaseNews/story?id=7192905&page=1
Magalski A. et al, St. Lukes Mid America Heart Institute Kansas.
- Aizer A. et al, Relation of vigorous exercise to atrial fibri., Am. J. of Card., 2009;103(11):1572-7.
- Gudmundsdottir S. et al, Physical activity and fertility in women, Hu. Repr. 2009; 0 :p337v1-dep337
- Madsen M. et al, Leisure time physical exercise during pregnancy and the risk of miscarriage, BR. J. Obs. Gyna. ; 114(11):1419-26.
- Sandmark H., Musculoskeletal dysfunction in phys. edu. teachers, Occup Envir Med 2000;57:673-7.
- Turner A. et al, Long term health impact of playing pro. football, Br J Sports Med 2000;34:332-6.
- Belda J. et al, Airway inflammation in the elite athlete, Br J Sports Med 2008;42:244-8.
- Bougault V. et al, Asthma airway inflammation and epithelial damage in swimmers and cold air athletes, Eur Respir J 2009;33:740-6.
- Intensive exercise is bad for your lungs, Melville K.,05-09-00.
www.scienceagogo.com/news/20000804223050data_trunc_sys.shtml
--------------------------------- Chapter 47 ---------------------------------
- Why exercise may not make you thin, Gray R., Telegraph, 24-08-09.
www.telegraph.co.uk/science/6083234/Health-warning-exercise-makes-you-fat.html
--------------------------------- Chapter 49 ---------------------------------
- Yoga helps asthma patients in ten weeks.
www.acsm.org/AM/Template.cfm?Section=ACSM_News_Releases&CONTENTID=12894&TEMPLATE=/CM/ContentDisplay.cfm
- Collet J. et al, The effects of Tai Chi on health outcomes in patients with chronic conditions, Arch Intern Med 2004;164:493-501.
- Hakin A. et al, Effects of walking on mortality among non-smoking retired men, New Eng J Med, 08-01-98 ;338(2):94-99.
- Richardson C. et a, Physical activity and mortality across cardiovascular disease groups, Med and Sci Sports and exercise, Nov 04; 36(11)1923-29.
- Weuve J. et al, Physical activity including walking and cognitive function in older women, JAMA 2004;292:1454-61.
- Abbott R. et al, Walking and dementia in physically capable older men, JAMA 2004;292:1447-53.
--------------------------------- Chapter 51 ---------------------------------
- Almeida O. et al, Low free testosterone concentration as a potentially treatable cause of depressive symptoms in older men, Arch Gen Psychiatry 2008;65(3):283-9.
- Laughlin G. et al, Low serum testosterone and mortality in older men, J Clin Endo and Metabolism 2008; 93(1):68-75.
- Parker W. et al, Ovarian conservation at the time of hysterectomy… , Obstetrics and Gynaecology May 2009;113(5):1027-37.
- Jensen T. et al, Good semen quality and life expectancy, Am J Epidemiology 2009;170(5):559-565.
--------------------------------- Chapter 54 ---------------------------------
- Sex Chemistry lasts two years, BBC, 01-02-06. http://news.bbc.co.uk/2/hi/4669104.stm
--------------------------------- Chapter 55 ---------------------------------
- Turek P. et al, Wet heat exposure, a potentially reversible cause of low semen quality in infertile men, Int Braz J Urol 2007; 33(1):50-6
- Mendiola J. et al, Food intake and its relationship with semen quality, Fertility and sterility March 2009 ; 91(3):812-8.
- Hamzelou J., If mum is happy and you know it, wave your fetal arms, New Scientist Magazine, 16-03-10,issue 2751.
- Wellcome Trust, 15-08-07, Eating junk food while pregnant and breastfeeding may lead to obese offspring.
- Stress harms brain in the womb, BBC,26-01-07. Glover V., http://news.bbc.co.uk/2/hi/6298909.stm
--------------------------------- Chapter 56 ---------------------------------
- Average UK woman wears 515 chemicals a day, Reuters, 19-11-09, Bionsen poll.
www.reuters.com/article/idUSTRE5AI3M820091119
--------------------------------- Chapter 58 ---------------------------------
- NHS in Numbers: then and now, BBC, 27-06-08. http://news.bbc.co.uk/2/hi/health/7475035.stm
- ICM Poll for Help The Aged, entitled Spotlight 2008.
- Chemical cosh for dementia kills 1800 a year, D. Rose, The Times, 13-11-09.
www.timesonline.co.uk/tol/life_and_style/health/article6914003.ece
--------------------------------- Chapter 59 ---------------------------------
- Tindle H. et al, Optimism, cynical hostility and incident coronary heart disease and mortality in the women's health initiative, Circulation, published online Aug 10-2009.
- Levy B. et al, Longevity increased by positive self perceptions of aging, J Personality and Soc. Pysch 2002 Aug; 83(2):261-70.
--------------------------------- Chapter 60 ---------------------------------
- Mercury in stream ecosystems, http://water.usgs.gov/nawqa/mercury/

Superior Health : The Secrets Of The Chinese And Eastern Way

- Schober S. et al, Blood mercury levels in US children and women of child bearing age, JAMA 2003 ;289(23):16671674.
- Zentek J. et al, Biological effects of transgenic maize NK603xMon810 fed inlong term reproduction studies in mice. Forschungberichte der sektion IV, Band 3, Institut fur ernahrung, and forchungs institut for biologist Landbau,Vienna, Austria Nov 08.
- Childrens Food Campaign 2008. www.childrensfoodcampaign.net/page4.htm
- Kaufman J. et al, Long term exposure to air pollution and incidence of cardiovascular events in women, New Eng J Med, Feb 2007; 356(5):447-458.
- Jerrett M. et al, Long term ozone exposure and mortality, New Eng J Med, 09; 360(11):1085-1095.
- Schier J. et al, Perchlorate exposure form infant formula and comparisons with the per chlorate reference dose, J Exposure Sci Environmental epidemiology 2010; 20:281-287.
- Jobling S. et al, Statistical modelling suggests that anti androgens in effluents from wastewater treatment works contribute to widespread sexual disruption in fish living in English rivers, Env Health Perspectives May 09; 117(5).
- Michels K. et al, Polycarbonate bottle use and urinary Bisphenol A concentrations, Env Health Perspectives 2009; 117 :1368-1372.
- Chunyuan Fei, Maternal levels of per fluorinated chemicals and sub fecundity, Human Reproduction, published online Jan 28 2009.
- Yao-Ping Lu et al, Tumorigenic effect of some commonly used moisturising creams when applied topically to UVB pre treated high risk mice , J Investigative Dermatology 2009; 129 :468-475.
- Corbel V. et al, Evidence for inhibition of cholinesterases in insect and mammalian nervous systems by the insect repellent Deet, BMC Biology 2009 ;7:47.
---------------------------------- Chapter 61 ----------------------------------
- More inequality in rich nations, BBC, 21-10-08, OECD '08, http://news.bbc.co.uk/2/hi/7681435.stm
- Virtanen M. et al, Long working hours and cognitive function, Am J epidemiology, online Jan 6 09.
- Nyberg A. et al, Managerial leadership and ischemic heart disease among employees, Occup Environ Med 2009;66:51-55.
- Chandola T. et al, Work stress and coronary heart disease : what are the mechanisms, European Heart Journal, online Jan 23 2008.
---------------------------------- Chapter 62 ----------------------------------
- NHS in Numbers: then and now, BBC, 27-06-08. http://news.bbc.co.uk/2/hi/health/7475035.stm
- Boyd W. et al, Insurance industry investments in tobacco, N Eng J Med June 2009;360(23):2483-84.
- Brenner D., Elliston C., Estimated Radiation risks potentially associated with full body CT screening, Radiology Sep 2004; 232:735-738.
- Brenner D., Hall E., Computed Tomography an increasing source of radiation exposure, N Eng J Med;357:2277-2284.
- Cambridge professor calls for healthy adults to use Ritalin to boost brain power, Daily Mail 10-12-08. www.dailymail.co.uk/health/article-1092826/Cambridge-professor-calls-healthy-adults-use-Ritalin-boost-brain-power.html
- Drugs don't work on many people, BBC, 08-12-03. http://news.bbc.co.uk/2/hi/3299945.stm
- Treating an illness is one thing. What about a patient with many, S. Carpenter, NY Times 30-03-09. www.nytimes.com/2009/03/31/health/31sick.html
- Drugs to reduce heart attack risks not working, R. Smith, Telegraph 01-11-09, Kotseva K. et al, www.telegraph.co.uk/health/healthnews/6117649/Drugs-to-reduce-heart-attack-risks-not-working.html
- Budnitz D. et al, Emergency department visits for antibiotics associated adverse events, Clinical Infectious Diseases 2008;47:735-743.
- Buchbinder R. et al, Randomized trial of vertebroplasty for painful osteoporotic vertebral fractures, New Eng J Med 2009; 361(6):557-568.
- Kallmes D. et al, Randomized trial of vertebroplasty for painful osteoporotic spinal fractures, New Eng J Med 2009; 361(6):569-579.
- Kirkley A. et al, A randomized trial of arthroscopic surgery for osteoarthritis of the knee, N Eng J Med 11-11-08; 359(11):1097-1107.
- Moseley J. et al, A controlled trial of arthroscopic surgery for osteoarthritis of the knee, N Eng J Med July 02; 347(2):81-88.
- Bhattacharya S. et al, Clomifene citrate or unstipulated intrauterine insemination compared with expectant management for unexplained infertility … , BMJ 2008 Aug 7;337:a716.
- www.britishfertilitysociety.org.uk/news/pressrelease/09_11-EggFreezinGuidelines.html
-Devereaux P. et al, Effects of extended release metropolis succinct in patients undergoing non cardiac surgery (POISE trial), Lancet 2008 May 31; 371 (9627):1839-47.
- Reimer C. et al, Proton pump inhibitor therapy induces acid related symptoms in healthy volunteers after withdrawal of therapy, Gastroenterology July 2009;137(1):80-87.
- Targownik L. et al, Use of proton pimp inhibitors and risk of osteoporosis relate fractures, CMAJ Aug 2008;179(4):319-26.

- Kirsch I. et al, Initial severity and antidepressant benefits: A meta analysis of data submitted to the FDA, PLOS Med 5(2):e45

---------------------------------- Chapter 63 ----------------------------------

- NHS safety failings kill 40,000 a year as patients pay price of target culture, Jenny Hope, Daily Mail 18-02-10, www.dailymail.co.uk/health/article-1251844/NHS-safety-failings-kill-40-000-year-patients-pay-price-target-culture.html

- Blundering hospitals kill 40,000 a year, Woolcock and Henderson, The Times 13-08-04, www.timesonline.co.uk/tol/news/uk/article468980.ece

- Starfield B., Is US health really the best in the world, JAMA 2000;284:483-485.

- Half of GPs refuse swine flu vaccine over testing fears, 25-08-09, www.dailymail.co.uk/news/article-1208716/Half-GPs-refuse-swine-flu-vaccine-testing-fears.html

---------------------------------- Chapter 65 ----------------------------------

- Nichol G. et al, regional variation in out of hospital cardiac arrest incidence and outcome, JAMA 2008;300(12):1423-1431.

- Surviving a heart attack, succumbing to heart failure, Gerald Couzens, New York Times, 29-01-09, http://health.nytimes.com/ref/health/healthguide/esn-heart-failure-ess.html

---------------------------------- Chapter 67 ----------------------------------

- Selfish adults damage childhood, BBC, 02-02-09, Mark Easton, The Good Children Inquiry, The Children's Society. http://news.bbc.co.uk/2/hi/uk_news/education/7861762.stm

- Twenge J. et al, Birth cohort increases in psychopathology in young Americans, 1938-2007: a cross temporal meta analysis of the MMPI, Clinical Psychology Review2010 ;30(2):145-54.

- More than 50% of college students felt suicidal, Sharon Jayson, USA Today, 18-08-08, www.usatoday.com/news/health/2008-08-17-college-suicidal-thoughts_N.htm

- Fuller-Thompson E., Brennenstuhl S., Making a link between childhood physical abuse and cancer: results from a regional representative survey , Cancer 2009; 115(14):3341-50.

- Sprehn G. et al, Decreased cancer survival in individuals separated at time of diagnosis, Cancer Aug 2009;115(21):5108-5116.

- Conzen S. et al, A model of gene environment interaction reveals mammary gland gene expression and increased tumor growth following social isolation, Cancer Prev Res Oct 2009;2(10):850-861.

-Kivipelto M. et al, Association between mid life marital status and cognitive function in later life: population based cohort study, BMJ 2009 Jul 2; 339:b2462.

-Wilson R. et al, Loneliness and risk of Alzheimer disease, Arch Gen Psych 2007; 64:234-240.

- Chandola T. et al, Negative aspects of close relationships and heart disease, Arch Intern Med 2007; 167(18):1951-1957.

- Satin J. et al, Depression as a predictor of disease mortality and progression in cancer patients, Cancer 2009; 115(22):5349-5361.

- Peled R. et al, Breast cancer, psychological distress and life events among young women, BMC Cancer 2008;8:245.

---------------------------------- Chapter 68 ----------------------------------

- Cohen S. et al, Emotional style and susceptibility to the common cold, Psychosomatic Med 65:652-657(2003).

- Davidson K. et al, Don't worry be happy: positive effect and reduced 10 year incident coronary heart disease: the Canadian Nova Scotia health study, Eur Heart J 2010; online Feb 17 2010.

- Giltay E. et al, Dispositional optimism and the risk of cardiovascular death: The Zutphen elderly study, Arch Intern Med 2006;166:431-466.

- Levy B. et al, longevity increased by positive self perceptions of aging, J Personality Social Psych Aug 2002;83(2).

- Maruta T. et al, Optimists Vs. Pessimists: survival rate among medical patients over a thirty year period, Mayo Clin Proc 2000;75:140-143.

---------------------------------- Chapter 70 ----------------------------------

- Ken Ho, Garvan Institute of Medical Research, Are the benefits of growth hormone in the athletes mind? , 25-06-08, www.garvan.org.au/news-events/news/are-the-benefits-of-growth-hormone-all-in-the-athletes-mind.html

- Benedetti F. et al, Placebo responsive Parkinson patients show decreased activity in single neurons of sub thalamic nucleus, Nature Neuroscience 2004; 7:587-588.

- Montgomery G. et al, A randomized clinical trial of a brief hypnosis intervention to control side effects in breast surgery patients, J Nat Can Inst 2007;99(17):1304-1312.

- Lang E. et al, Adjunctive non pharmacological analgesia for invasive medical procedures: a randomized trial, Lancet April 2000;355(9214):1486-1490.

- Woman lost 4stone after hypnotist convinced her of gastric band fitting, Telegraph 20-05-09. www.telegraph.co.uk/news/uknews/5357013/Woman-lost-4st-after-hypnotist-convinced-her-of-gastric-band-fitting.html

- Placebo effects shocks allergy drugs maker, BBC News, 05-07-99. http://news.bbc.co.uk/2/hi/business/386773.stm

- Tilburt J. et al, Prescribing placebo treatments: results of national survey of US internists and rheumatologists, BMJ 2008; 337:a1938.

Selected Bibliography.

The Foundations of Chinese Medicine - Giovanni Maciocia, Churchill Livingstone.
The Practice of Chinese Medicine - Giovanni Maciocia, Churchill Livingstone.
Clinical Medicine - Parveen Kumar and Michael Clark, W.B.Saunders.
Healing With Whole Foods, Asian Traditions And Modern Nutrition - Paul Pitchford, North Atlantic.
The Essential Book Of Traditional Chinese Medicine Volume 1 Theory - Liu Yanchi, Columbia.
The Essential Book Of Traditional Chinese Medicine Volume 2 Clinical - Liu Yanchi, Columbia.
The Tao Of Healthy Eating - Bob Flaws, Blue Poppy Press.
Chinese Medical Qigong Therapy - Dr. Jerry Alan Johnson, International Institute Medical Qigong.
The Tao Of Nutrition - Maoshing Ni with Cathy McNease, Seven Star Communications.
Chinese Natural Cures - Henry C.Lu, Black Dog And Leventhal Publishers.
The Tao And The Tree Of Life - Eric Steven Yudelove, Llewellyn Publications.
Chinese Medicine - Ted J. Kaptchuk, Rider Books.
A Complete Guide To Chi Gung - Daniel Reid, Shambhala.
Secrets Of Longevity - Maoshing Ni, Chronicle Books.
Scholar Warrior - Deng Ming-Dao, Harper One.
Healthy At 100 - John Robbins, Ballantine Books.
5 Secrets Of Health And Happiness - Angela Hicks, Thorsons.
Meditation For Busy People - Osho, St. Martins Griffin.
Love And Survival - Dr. Dean Ornish, Vermilion.
The Complete Book Of Chinese Medicine - Wong Kiew Kit, Cosmos.
Traditional Chinese Medicine For women - Xiaolan Zhao, Virago.
The China Study - T. Colin Campbell and Thomas M. Campbell II, Benbella.
The Body Electric - Robert O. Becker and Gary Selden, Harper.
The Roots Of Chinese Qigong - Dr. Yang Jwing-Ming, YMAA Publication Centre.
The Yellow Emperor's Classic Of Medicine - Maoshing Ni, Shambhala.
The Tao Of Health, Sex And Longevity - Daniel Reid, Simon And Schuster.
Japanese Women Don't Get Old Or Fat - Naomi Moriyama, Vermilion.
The Biology Of Belief - Bruce H.Lipton, Mountain Of Love / Elite Books.
The Merck Manual Of Medical Information - Robert Berkow, Pocket Books.
Death By Modern Medicine - Dr.Carolyn Dean And Trueman Tuck, Matrix Verite.
The Power Of Your Subconscious Mind - Dr. Joseph Murphy, Pocket Books.
Modern Medicine: The New World Religion - Oliver Clerc, Personhood Press.
Hippocrates Shadow - David H. Newman, Scribner.
Transform Stress Into Vitality - Mantak Chia, Healing Tao Books.
What Doctors Don't Tell You - Lynne McTaggart, Thorsons.

Acknowledgements.

Grateful thanks to Karen Powell, Peter Young, Robert Hughes, Carl and Jean Wray who all provided help during the editing of this book.

Thanks to Eleanor Hopkins for providing the illustration on page 222.

And heartfelt thanks to all the great scientists, philosophers and gurus, doctors and healers, past and present who have devoted their lives to trying to make a better, healthier and happier world for us all to share and live in.

Lightning Source UK Ltd.
Milton Keynes UK
13 November 2010

162806UK00002B/2/P